FATTY LIVER DIET FOOD LIST

Thrive Every Day: A 30-Day Meal Plan for Vibrant Health

Dr Angela Sorrell

Copyright © 2024

All Rights Are Reserved

The content in this book may not be reproduced, duplicated, or transferred without the express written permission of the author or publisher. Under no circumstances will the publisher or author be held liable or legally responsible for any losses, expenditures, or damages incurred directly or indirectly as a consequence of the information included in this book.

Legal Remarks

Copyright protection applies to this publication. It is only intended for personal use. No piece of this work may be modified, distributed, sold, quoted, or paraphrased without the author's or publisher's consent.

Disclaimer Statement

Please keep in mind that the contents of this booklet are meant for educational and recreational purposes. Every effort has been made to offer accurate, up-to-date, reliable, and thorough information. There are, however, no stated or implied assurances of any kind. Readers understand that the author is providing competent counsel. The content in this book originates from several sources. Please seek the opinion of a competent professional before using any of the tactics outlined in this book. By reading this book, the reader agrees that the author will not be held accountable for any direct or indirect damages resulting from the use of the information contained therein, including, but not limited to, errors, omissions, or inaccuracies.

Table of Contents

Table of Contents

INTRODUCTION

Hey there, fellow foodies and liver warriors!

If you're holding this book, chances are you've stumbled upon that pesky diagnosis: "Fatty Liver Disease." Maybe your doctor dropped the bombshell during a routine checkup, or perhaps you've been grappling with the symptoms for a while now, wondering what the heck is going on with your body.

First off, let me extend a virtual hug your way. *Hug* I know, getting hit with a diagnosis like fatty liver can feel like a punch in the gut. Suddenly, your favorite foods become suspect, and you're left wondering if your liver is secretly plotting against you.

But fear not, my friend! This book is your beacon of hope in the sea of dietary confusion. Consider it your trusty sidekick on the journey to reclaiming your liver health and your taste buds!

Now, before we dive headfirst into the tantalizing world of food lists and liver-loving recipes, let's address the elephant in the room: Fatty Liver Disease. It's not exactly the glamorous disease du jour, is it? I mean, you won't find Instagram influencers flaunting their latest liver-friendly smoothie bowl recipe. But hey, who needs Instar-fame when you've got a liver that's begging for some TLC?

In these pages, we'll unpack the mysteries of fatty liver disease together. We'll chat about why our livers sometimes decide to throw a temper tantrum, what foods make them happy, and which ones send them into a tailspin. Think of it as a crash course in Liver 101, minus the boring lectures and pop quizzes.

But let's get one thing straight from the get-go: I'm not here to preach from some ivory tower of perfect health. Nope, I'm right here in the trenches with you, armed with a spatula and a healthy dose of empathy. I get it. I understand the frustration of flipping through endless internet articles, each one spouting conflicting advice about what to eat and what to avoid.

That's why I've crafted this book with you in mind, dear reader. I've sifted through the mountains of nutritional jargon and boiled it down to the good stuff – pun intended. You won't find any pretentious chef-speak or impossible-to-pronounce ingredients here. Just practical, down-to-earth guidance to help you navigate the choppy waters of fatty liver management.

So, what can you expect from these pages? Well, consider it your culinary roadmap to liver health. We'll start by laying the groundwork with a crash course on fatty liver disease – think of it as Liver 101, but with fewer snooze-worthy lectures and wittier banter.

Then, we'll roll up our sleeves and dive into the heart of the matter: The Fatty Liver Diet Food List. Spoiler alert: it's not as restrictive as you might think! We'll explore a smorgasbord of lean proteins, healthy fats, and fiber-rich goodies that'll have your taste buds doing a happy dance.

But fear not, my friend! This book is your beacon of hope in the sea of dietary confusion. Consider it your trusty sidekick on the journey to reclaiming your liver health and your taste buds!

Now, before we dive headfirst into the tantalizing world of food lists and liver-loving recipes, let's address the elephant in the room: Fatty Liver Disease. It's not exactly the glamorous disease du jour, is it? I mean, you won't find Instagram influencers flaunting their latest liver-friendly smoothie bowl recipe. But hey, who needs Instar-fame when you've got a liver that's begging for some TLC?

In these pages, we'll unpack the mysteries of fatty liver disease together. We'll chat about why our livers sometimes decide to throw a temper tantrum, what foods make them happy, and which ones send them into a tailspin. Think of it as a crash course in Liver 101, minus the boring lectures and pop quizzes.

But let's get one thing straight from the get-go: I'm not here to preach from some ivory tower of perfect health. Nope, I'm right here in the trenches with you, armed with a spatula and a healthy dose of empathy. I get it. I understand the frustration of flipping through endless internet articles, each one spouting conflicting advice about what to eat and what to avoid.

That's why I've crafted this book with you in mind, dear reader. I've sifted through the mountains of nutritional jargon and boiled it down to the good stuff – pun intended. You won't find any pretentious chef-speak or impossible-to-pronounce ingredients here. Just practical, down-to-earth guidance to help you navigate the choppy waters of fatty liver management.

So, what can you expect from these pages? Well, consider it your culinary roadmap to liver health. We'll start by laying the groundwork with a crash course on fatty liver disease – think of it as Liver 101, but with fewer snooze-worthy lectures and wittier banter.

Then, we'll roll up our sleeves and dive into the heart of the matter: The Fatty Liver Diet Food List. Spoiler alert: it's not as restrictive as you might think! We'll explore a smorgasbord of lean proteins, healthy fats, and fiber-rich goodies that'll have your taste buds doing a happy dance. But wait, there's more! We'll also dish out some handy tips for meal planning, share mouthwatering recipes that even the most novice chef can master, and sprinkle in a healthy dose of humor along the way. After all, laughter is the best medicine – well, that and a heaping plate of liver-friendly grub.

So, whether you're a seasoned health nut or a culinary newbie, grab a fork and join me on this delicious journey to liver wellness. Together, we'll whip up some tasty dishes, banish those liver woes, and maybe – just maybe – have a little fun along the way.

Let's do this!

Warmest regards,

CHAPTER ONE

THE FATTY LIVER DIET APPROACH

Fatty liver disease, characterized by an excess accumulation of fat in the liver cells, has become increasingly prevalent in recent years. While genetics and other factors play a role, diet is a key component in the development and management of this condition. In this chapter, we'll explore the principles of a fatty liver diet and the benefits of following such an approach.

Principles of a Fatty Liver Diet

When it comes to managing fatty liver disease through diet, the overarching goal is to reduce liver fat accumulation, alleviate inflammation, and promote overall liver health. To achieve these objectives, certain dietary principles should be followed:

- **Limit Saturated and Trans Fats**: Saturated fats, found in foods like red meat, butter, and full-fat dairy products, as well as trans fats found in processed and fried foods, can contribute to liver inflammation and worsen fatty liver disease. Therefore, it's essential to minimize the intake of these fats in the diet. Instead, opt for healthier sources of fat such as avocados, nuts, seeds, and olive oil.

- **Emphasize Healthy Fats**: Not all fats are created equal. Healthy fats, such as monounsaturated and polyunsaturated fats, play a crucial role in reducing inflammation and supporting liver function. Foods rich in these fats include fatty fish like salmon and mackerel, avocados, nuts, and seeds. Incorporating these fats into your diet can help improve liver health and reduce the risk of complications associated with fatty liver disease.

- **Choose Complex Carbohydrates**: Simple carbohydrates like refined sugars and white flour can spike blood sugar levels and contribute to liver fat accumulation. In contrast, complex carbohydrates, found in whole grains, fruits, and vegetables, provide a steady source of energy and fiber without causing sharp increases in blood sugar. These foods should form the foundation of a fatty liver diet, helping to maintain stable blood sugar levels and promote satiety.

- **Prioritize Lean Protein**: Protein is an essential nutrient for liver health, as it plays a crucial role in repairing liver cells and supporting detoxification processes. However, not all sources of protein are created equal. Opt for lean protein sources such as poultry, fish, tofu, beans, and legumes, which are lower in saturated fat and beneficial for overall health. Limiting the intake of red meat and processed meats can help reduce inflammation and improve liver function.

- **Increase Fiber Intake**: Dietary fiber is known for its role in promoting digestive health, but it also plays a vital role in managing fatty liver disease. Fiber helps to regulate blood sugar levels, promote satiety, and support healthy digestion, all of which are important for liver health. Incorporate plenty of fiber-rich foods such as fruits, vegetables, whole grains, and legumes into your diet to support liver function and reduce inflammation.

- **Moderate Alcohol Consumption**: Excessive alcohol consumption is a leading cause of fatty liver disease and can exacerbate existing liver damage. If you have fatty liver disease, it's essential to limit alcohol intake or avoid it altogether. Even moderate alcohol consumption can contribute to liver inflammation and worsen the condition. Instead, opt for non-alcoholic beverages such as water, herbal tea, or sparkling water flavored with fresh fruit.

- **Stay Hydrated**: Proper hydration is essential for liver health, as it helps flush toxins from the body and supports overall liver function. Aim to drink plenty of water throughout the day to stay hydrated and support optimal liver health. Limiting sugary beverages and opting for water, herbal tea, or infused water can help reduce liver fat accumulation and promote overall well-being.

Following these principles can help reduce liver fat accumulation, alleviate inflammation, and improve overall liver health. However, it's essential to tailor your diet to your individual needs and consult with a healthcare professional or registered dietitian for personalized recommendations.

Benefits of Following a Fatty Liver Diet

Now that we've covered the principles of a fatty liver diet, let's explore the benefits of following such an approach:

- **Improved Liver Function**: By reducing liver fat accumulation and inflammation, a fatty liver diet can help improve liver function and prevent further damage. Incorporating nutrient-rich foods and limiting harmful substances such as alcohol and unhealthy fats can support optimal liver health and function.

- **Reduced Risk of Complications**: Fatty liver disease is associated with an increased risk of complications such as liver cirrhosis, liver cancer, and cardiovascular disease. Following a fatty liver diet can help reduce these risks by promoting liver health, managing inflammation, and improving overall well-being.

- **Weight Management**: Many individuals with fatty liver disease are overweight or obese, which can exacerbate the condition. A fatty liver diet emphasizes nutrient-dense, whole foods and encourages portion control, which can support weight loss or weight management goals. By maintaining a healthy weight, individuals can reduce the strain on their liver and improve their overall health.

- **Better Blood Sugar Control**: Stable blood sugar levels are essential for managing fatty liver disease, as fluctuations in blood sugar can contribute to liver fat accumulation and inflammation. The complex carbohydrates and fiber-rich foods emphasized in a fatty liver diet can help regulate blood sugar levels and reduce the risk of complications associated with diabetes and fatty liver disease.

- **Increased Energy and Vitality**: Eating a nutritious diet can help increase energy levels, improve mood, and enhance overall vitality. By fueling the body with nutrient-rich foods and supporting liver health, individuals may experience improved energy levels, mental clarity, and overall well-being.

- **Long-Term Health Benefits**: Adopting a fatty liver diet isn't just about managing the symptoms of fatty liver disease; it's about promoting long-term health and well-being. By making positive changes to your diet and lifestyle, you can reduce your risk of developing chronic diseases such as diabetes, heart disease, and certain types of cancer.

CHAPTER TWO

ESSENTIAL NUTRIENTS FOR FATTY LIVER HEALTH

In the realm of managing fatty liver disease, paying attention to nutrient intake is paramount. The foods we consume play a significant role not only in fueling our bodies but also in supporting liver health and function. In this chapter, we'll delve into the importance of nutrient-rich foods and explore key nutrients essential for maintaining optimal liver health.

Importance of Nutrient-Rich Foods

Nutrient-rich foods are those that are packed with essential vitamins, minerals, antioxidants, and other compounds that are vital for overall health and well-being. When it comes to fatty liver disease, focusing on nutrient-rich foods is especially important, as these foods can help reduce inflammation, support liver function, and promote overall wellness.

One of the primary benefits of nutrient-rich foods is their ability to provide the body with the nutrients it needs to function optimally. Essential vitamins and minerals such as vitamin C, vitamin E, selenium, and zinc play crucial roles in supporting liver health by acting as antioxidants, helping to neutralize harmful free radicals, and reducing oxidative stress.

Additionally, nutrient-rich foods are often high in fiber, which is beneficial for digestive health and can help regulate blood sugar levels. High-fiber foods such as fruits, vegetables, whole grains, and legumes can help promote satiety, prevent overeating, and support weight management – all of which are important considerations for individuals with fatty liver disease.

Furthermore, nutrient-rich foods are typically lower in unhealthy fats, sugars, and processed ingredients, which can contribute to liver fat accumulation and inflammation. By choosing nutrient-rich foods over processed and unhealthy options, individuals can reduce their risk of developing or exacerbating fatty liver disease.

Overall, incorporating a variety of nutrient-rich foods into the diet is essential for supporting liver health, reducing inflammation, and promoting overall well-being. By focusing on whole, minimally processed foods rich in vitamins, minerals, and antioxidants, individuals can take proactive steps to manage fatty liver disease and improve their quality of life.

Key Nutrients for Liver Health

Now that we understand the importance of nutrient-rich foods, let's explore some key nutrients that are particularly beneficial for liver health:

- **Omega-3 Fatty Acids**: Omega-3 fatty acids are a type of healthy fat found in fatty fish such as salmon, mackerel, and sardines, as well as in walnuts, flaxseeds, and chia seeds. These essential fatty acids have been shown to reduce inflammation, improve liver function, and decrease liver fat accumulation. Incorporating omega-3-rich foods into the diet can help support liver health and reduce the risk of complications associated with fatty liver disease.

- **Antioxidants**: Antioxidants are compounds that help protect the body from oxidative stress and damage caused by free radicals. Vitamins C and E, selenium, and zinc are all powerful antioxidants that play crucial roles in supporting liver health. Foods rich in antioxidants include fruits, vegetables, nuts, seeds, and whole grains. By incorporating these foods into the diet, individuals can help reduce inflammation, support liver function, and promote overall well-being.

- **B Vitamins**: B vitamins, including folate, B6, and B12, are essential for liver health and function. These vitamins play key roles in energy metabolism, DNA synthesis, and the production of red blood cells. Foods rich in B vitamins include leafy greens, legumes, whole grains, eggs, and lean meats. Ensuring an adequate intake of B vitamins is important for supporting liver health and preventing deficiencies that can contribute to liver dysfunction.

- **Vitamin D**: Vitamin D is a fat-soluble vitamin that plays a crucial role in immune function, bone health, and overall well-being. Recent research has also suggested that vitamin D may play a role in liver health, with low levels of vitamin D being associated with an increased risk of fatty liver disease. Foods rich in vitamin D include fatty fish, fortified dairy products, and fortified cereals. Additionally, exposure to sunlight can stimulate the body's production of vitamin D. Ensuring adequate vitamin D intake through diet and sunlight exposure is important for supporting liver health and overall well-being.

- **Choline**: Choline is an essential nutrient that plays a key role in liver health and fat metabolism. Choline is involved in the synthesis of phospholipids, which are essential components of cell membranes and are involved in fat transport and metabolism. Foods rich in choline include eggs, liver, lean meats, and cruciferous vegetables such as broccoli and Brussels sprouts. Ensuring an adequate intake of choline is important for supporting liver health and preventing deficiencies that can contribute to fatty liver disease.

CHAPTER THREE

FATTY LIVER DIET FOOD LIST

In the journey towards managing fatty liver disease, one of the most crucial components is the diet. What you eat can either exacerbate the condition or support your liver health and aid in its recovery. In this comprehensive guide, we'll explore a variety of foods that are beneficial for individuals with fatty liver disease, categorized into different groups to simplify your dietary choices.

Lean Protein Sources

Protein is an essential nutrient for liver health, as it plays a crucial role in repairing liver cells and supporting detoxification processes. However, not all protein sources are created equal, especially for individuals with fatty liver disease. Lean protein sources are preferred as they contain less saturated fat and are less likely to contribute to liver inflammation. Here are some excellent options:

- **Chicken Breast**: Skinless, boneless chicken breast is a fantastic lean protein source. It's versatile, easy to cook, and low in fat. A 3-ounce serving of grilled chicken breast provides around 165 calories, 31 grams of protein, and only 3.6 grams of fat.

- **Turkey Breast**: Similarly, turkey breast is another lean protein option that's low in fat and high in protein. It's a great alternative to chicken and can be used in various recipes. A 3-ounce serving of roasted turkey breast contains approximately 125 calories, 26 grams of protein, and only 1.5 grams of fat.

- **Fish**: Fatty fish like salmon, mackerel, and sardines are rich in omega-3 fatty acids, which have anti-inflammatory properties and are beneficial for liver health. These fish also provide high-quality protein without excessive saturated fat. A 3-ounce serving of salmon, for example, provides around 177 calories, 23 grams of protein, and 9.8 grams of fat.

- **Tofu**: For vegetarian or vegan options, tofu is an excellent source of plant-based protein. It's low in fat and can be used in a variety of dishes, from stir-fries to salads. A 3-ounce serving of tofu contains approximately 70 calories, 8 grams of protein, and 4 grams of fat.

- **Legumes**: Beans, lentils, and chickpeas are nutrient-dense sources of protein that are also high in fiber. They provide sustained energy and can help stabilize blood sugar levels. A 1/2 cup serving of cooked lentils, for example, contains around 115 calories, 9 grams of protein, and only 0.4 grams of fat.

Incorporating lean protein sources into your diet can help support liver health and provide essential nutrients without contributing to liver fat accumulation or inflammation. Aim to include a variety of these foods in your meals to ensure you're getting a well-rounded intake of protein while managing fatty liver disease.

Healthy Fats and Oils

Contrary to popular belief, not all fats are bad for you – in fact, some fats are essential for overall health, including liver health. Healthy fats are an essential component of a balanced diet, and they play a crucial role in supporting cell structure, hormone production, and nutrient absorption.

When it comes to fatty liver disease, choosing the right fats and oils is key. Here are some healthy options to consider:

- **Olive Oil**: Extra virgin olive oil is a staple of Mediterranean cuisine and is renowned for its health benefits. It's rich in monounsaturated fats and contains powerful antioxidants that have anti-inflammatory properties. Use olive oil for cooking, salad dressings, and marinades to add flavor and nutrition to your meals.

- **Avocado**: Avocado is a unique fruit that's rich in healthy fats, particularly monounsaturated fats. It's also packed with fiber, vitamins, and minerals, making it a nutritious addition to any diet. Enjoy avocado sliced on toast, blended into smoothies, or mashed into guacamole for a tasty and satisfying treat.

- **Nuts and Seeds**: Almonds, walnuts, flaxseeds, chia seeds, and hemp seeds are all excellent sources of healthy fats, protein, and fiber. They're perfect for snacking or adding crunch to salads, yogurt, or oatmeal. Just be mindful of portion sizes, as nuts and seeds are calorie-dense foods.

- **Fatty Fish**: As mentioned earlier, fatty fish like salmon, mackerel, and sardines are rich in omega-3 fatty acids, which are highly beneficial for liver health. Aim to include fatty fish in your diet at least twice a week to reap the benefits of their healthy fats.

- **Coconut Oil**: While controversial, coconut oil has gained popularity in recent years for its potential health benefits. It contains medium-chain triglycerides (MCTs), which are a type of saturated fat that is metabolized differently in the body compared to other fats. Some studies suggest that coconut oil may have anti-inflammatory and liver-protective effects, but more research is needed to confirm these findings. Use coconut oil sparingly and opt for virgin or unrefined varieties for the most nutritional benefits.

It's essential to include healthy fats in your diet to support liver health and overall well-being. By choosing sources like olive oil, avocado, nuts, seeds, and fatty fish, you can provide your body with the essential fatty acids it needs while managing fatty liver disease.

Fiber-Rich Foods

Fiber is a nutrient that's often overlooked but plays a crucial role in supporting digestive health, regulating blood sugar levels, and promoting satiety. For individuals with fatty liver disease, incorporating fiber-rich foods into the diet is especially important, as fiber can help reduce liver fat accumulation and improve insulin sensitivity. Here are some fiber-rich foods to include in your diet:

- **Fruits**: Berries, apples, pears, oranges, and bananas are all excellent sources of dietary fiber. They're also rich in vitamins, minerals, and antioxidants, making them a nutritious choice for snacks or desserts. Aim to eat a variety of fruits to get the most nutritional benefits.

- **Vegetables**: Leafy greens like spinach, kale, and Swiss chard are packed with fiber and essential nutrients. Other fiber-rich vegetables include broccoli, Brussels sprouts, carrots, and sweet potatoes. Incorporate a variety of colorful vegetables into your meals to maximize your fiber intake and support liver health.

- **Whole Grains**: Whole grains like oats, quinoa, brown rice, and barley are excellent sources of fiber and complex carbohydrates. They provide sustained energy and can help stabilize blood sugar levels, which is important for managing fatty liver disease. Replace refined grains with whole grains whenever possible to increase your fiber intake and improve overall nutrition.

- **Legumes**: Beans, lentils, and chickpeas are all high in fiber and protein, making them a nutritious addition to any diet. They're also low in fat and cholesterol-free, making them heart-healthy choices. Add legumes to soups, stews, salads, and stir-fries to increase your fiber intake and support liver health.

- **Nuts and Seeds**: In addition to healthy fats, nuts and seeds are also rich in fiber. Almonds, walnuts, flaxseeds, chia seeds, and hemp seeds are all excellent choices for increasing your fiber intake. Enjoy them as snacks, sprinkle them on salads or yogurt, or use them in baking to add texture and flavor to your favorite recipes.

Increasing your fiber intake is an essential part of managing fatty liver disease and supporting overall health. By incorporating fiber-rich foods like fruits, vegetables, whole grains, legumes, nuts, and seeds into your diet, you can improve digestion, regulate blood sugar levels, and promote liver health.

Low-Glycemic Index Carbohydrates

Carbohydrates often get a bad rap, but not all carbs are created equal. The glycemic index (GI) is a measure of how quickly a carbohydrate-containing food raises blood sugar levels. Foods with a low GI are digested and absorbed more slowly, leading to gradual increases in blood sugar levels and providing sustained energy. For individuals with fatty liver disease, choosing low-GI carbohydrates can help stabilize blood sugar levels and reduce the risk of complications. Here are some examples of low-GI carbohydrates to include in your diet:

- **Whole Grains**: Whole grains like oats, quinoa, barley, and brown rice have a lower GI compared to refined grains like white bread, white rice, and pasta. They're also high in fiber, vitamins, and minerals, making them a nutritious choice for meals and snacks.

- **Legumes**: Beans, lentils, and chickpeas are all low-GI carbohydrates that are also rich in fiber and protein. They provide sustained energy and can help stabilize blood sugar levels, making them an excellent choice for individuals with fatty liver disease.

- **Non-Starchy Vegetables**: Vegetables like broccoli, cauliflower, spinach, kale, and bell peppers are low in calories and carbohydrates but high in fiber, vitamins, and minerals. They have a minimal impact on blood sugar levels and can be enjoyed in large quantities as part of a healthy diet.

- **Sweet Potatoes**: Unlike white potatoes, which have a higher GI, sweet potatoes have a lower GI and are packed with fiber, vitamins, and antioxidants. They're a nutritious and delicious alternative to traditional potatoes and can be enjoyed roasted, mashed, or baked.

- **Berries**: Berries like strawberries, blueberries, raspberries, and blackberries are low in calories and carbohydrates but high in fiber and antioxidants. They're a sweet and satisfying snack that won't cause spikes in blood sugar levels.

Choosing low-GI carbohydrates can help stabilize blood sugar levels, reduce the risk of complications, and promote overall health and well-being. By incorporating whole grains, legumes, non-starchy vegetables, sweet potatoes, and berries into your diet, you can support liver health and manage fatty liver disease more effectively.

Antioxidant-Rich Fruits and Vegetables

Antioxidants are compounds that help protect the body from oxidative stress and damage caused by free radicals. They play a crucial role in reducing inflammation, supporting immune function, and promoting overall health and well-being. For individuals with fatty liver disease, incorporating antioxidant-rich fruits and vegetables into the diet is essential for supporting liver health and reducing the risk of complications. Here are some antioxidant-rich foods to include in your diet:

- **Berries**: Berries like strawberries, blueberries, raspberries, and blackberries are packed with antioxidants, including vitamin C, flavonoids, and polyphenols. These compounds have anti-inflammatory properties and can help protect liver cells from damage caused by oxidative stress.

- **Leafy Greens**: Dark, leafy greens like spinach, kale, Swiss chard, and collard greens are rich in antioxidants, vitamins, and minerals. They're also high in fiber, which is beneficial for digestion and overall health. Incorporate a variety of leafy greens into your meals to maximize your antioxidant intake and support liver health.

- **Cruciferous Vegetables**: Vegetables like broccoli, Brussels sprouts, cauliflower, and cabbage are packed with antioxidants and sulfur compounds that have liver-protective effects. They also contain fiber, which can help reduce cholesterol levels and improve digestion.

- **Citrus Fruits**: Citrus fruits like oranges, lemons, limes, and grapefruits are rich in vitamin C, a powerful antioxidant that helps neutralize free radicals and support immune function. Enjoy citrus fruits as snacks, in salads, or as part of your favorite recipes to boost your antioxidant intake and promote liver health.

- **Tomatoes**: Tomatoes are an excellent source of lycopene, a potent antioxidant that has been shown to have liver-protective effects. They're also rich in vitamins A and C, as well as other beneficial compounds like beta-carotene and lutein. Enjoy tomatoes fresh in salads, soups, or sandwiches, or cook them into sauces, stews, and casseroles.

Incorporating antioxidant-rich fruits and vegetables into your diet is essential for supporting liver health, reducing inflammation, and promoting overall well-being. By including a variety of colorful fruits and vegetables in your meals, you can ensure you're getting a wide range of antioxidants and other essential nutrients to support your liver and improve your health.

Beverages for Liver Health

When it comes to liver health, what you drink is just as important as what you eat. Beverages can have a significant impact on liver function, inflammation, and overall well-being. For individuals with fatty liver disease, choosing the right beverages can help support liver health and aid in the management of the condition. Here are some beverages to consider incorporating into your diet:

- **Water**: Staying hydrated is essential for liver health, as it helps flush toxins from the body and supports overall liver function. Aim to drink at least eight glasses of water per day, and more if you're active or live in a hot climate. Water is the best choice for hydration, as it contains zero calories and no added sugars.

- **Herbal Tea**: Herbal teas like green tea, dandelion tea, and milk thistle tea are rich in antioxidants and have liver-protective effects. Green tea, in particular, contains catechism, which have been shown to reduce liver fat accumulation and improve liver function. Enjoy herbal teas hot or cold as a refreshing and healthful beverage option.

- **Vegetable Juice**: Freshly squeezed vegetable juices are a nutritious way to hydrate and support liver health. Vegetables like carrots, beets, celery, and kale are rich in vitamins, minerals, and antioxidants that can help reduce inflammation and support detoxification processes. Blend up your favorite combination of vegetables for a tasty and nutritious beverage.

- **Fruit Smoothies**: Fruit smoothies made with antioxidant-rich fruits like berries, citrus fruits, and tropical fruits can provide a delicious and nutritious way to support liver health. Use unsweetened almond milk or coconut water as a base and add in your favorite fruits for flavor and nutrition. Avoid adding excessive amounts of sugar or sweeteners to keep your smoothies healthful.

- **Water with Lemon**: Starting your day with a glass of water with lemon can help stimulate digestion, support liver function, and promote detoxification. Lemon water is alkalizing and can help balance the body's pH levels, which is beneficial for overall health. Squeeze half a lemon into a glass of water and enjoy it first thing in the morning for a refreshing and healthful beverage.

Incorporating these beverages into your daily routine can help support liver health, reduce inflammation, and promote overall well-being. By choosing hydrating, antioxidant-rich options like water, herbal tea, vegetable juice, fruit smoothies, and lemon water, you can give your liver the support it needs to function optimally and improve your health.

CHAPTER FOUR

FOODS TO AVOID FOR FATTY LIVER

In the battle against fatty liver disease, knowing which foods to avoid is just as important as knowing which foods to include in your diet. Certain dietary choices can exacerbate liver inflammation, contribute to liver fat accumulation, and increase the risk of complications associated with the condition. In this chapter, we'll explore four categories of foods to avoid for fatty liver disease and discuss why they should be limited or eliminated from your diet.

High-Fat Foods

High-fat foods, especially those high in saturated and trans fats, should be limited in a fatty liver diet. These fats can contribute to liver fat accumulation, increase inflammation, and worsen insulin resistance, all of which can exacerbate fatty liver disease. Here are some high-fat foods to avoid or limit in your diet:

- **Fried Foods**: Fried foods like French fries, fried chicken, and onion rings are loaded with unhealthy fats and calories. They're often cooked in hydrogenated oils, which are high in trans fats – the worst type of fat for liver health. Consuming fried foods regularly can contribute to liver inflammation and increase the risk of complications associated with fatty liver disease.

- **Processed Meats**: Processed meats like bacon, sausage, hot dogs, and deli meats are high in saturated fat, cholesterol, and sodium. They're also often treated with nitrates and other preservatives, which can be harmful to liver health. Limiting or avoiding processed meats can help reduce your intake of unhealthy fats and lower your risk of fatty liver disease.

- **Fast Food**: Fast food items like burgers, pizza, and tacos are typically high in saturated and trans fats, as well as sodium and added sugars. They're also calorie-dense and nutrient-poor, meaning they provide little nutritional value while contributing to weight gain and liver fat accumulation. Limiting your intake of fast food can help improve liver health and overall well-being.

- **Full-Fat Dairy Products**: Full-fat dairy products like whole milk, cheese, and butter are high in saturated fat, which can contribute to liver fat accumulation and inflammation. Opt for low-fat or fat-free dairy alternatives, such as skim milk, reduced-fat cheese, and yogurt, to reduce your intake of unhealthy fats and support liver health.

- **Baked Goods**: Baked goods like pastries, cakes, cookies, and doughnuts are often made with refined flour, sugar, and unhealthy fats. They're calorie-dense and nutrient-poor, and consuming them regularly can contribute to liver fat accumulation and insulin resistance. Limiting your intake of baked goods and opting for healthier alternatives like whole grain bread, oatmeal cookies, and homemade muffins can help support liver health.

By limiting your intake of high-fat foods like fried foods, processed meats, fast food, full-fat dairy products, and baked goods, you can reduce your risk of liver fat accumulation, inflammation, and complications associated with fatty liver disease. Instead, focus on incorporating nutrient-rich, whole foods into your diet to support liver health and overall well-being.

Sugary Foods and Beverages

Excessive sugar consumption is strongly linked to fatty liver disease and can contribute to liver fat accumulation, insulin resistance, and inflammation. Sugary foods and beverages should be limited or avoided in a fatty liver diet to reduce the risk of complications and support liver health. Here are some sugary foods and beverages to avoid or limit in your diet:

- **Soda and Sweetened Beverages**: Soda, fruit juice, energy drinks, sweetened teas, and sports drinks are all high in added sugars, which can contribute to liver fat accumulation and insulin resistance. Drinking these beverages regularly can increase the risk of fatty liver disease and other metabolic conditions. Opt for water, herbal tea, or unsweetened beverages instead to support liver health.

- **Candy and Sweets**: Candy, chocolate, cookies, cakes, and other sweet treats are high in sugar and calories and provide little nutritional value. Consuming these foods regularly can lead to weight gain, liver fat accumulation, and insulin resistance. Limit your intake of sweets and opt for healthier alternatives like fresh fruit, yogurt, or dark chocolate with a high cocoa content.

- **Processed Snacks**: Processed snacks like chips, crackers, granola bars, and snack cakes are often high in added sugars, refined carbohydrates, and unhealthy fats. They're calorie-dense and nutrient-poor, and consuming them regularly can contribute to liver fat accumulation and inflammation. Choose healthier snack options like fresh fruit, nuts, seeds, or whole grain crackers to support liver health.

- **Sweetened Condiments**: Condiments like ketchup, barbecue sauce, teriyaki sauce, and salad dressings often contain added sugars and unhealthy fats. Using these condiments liberally can increase your overall sugar intake and contribute to liver fat accumulation. Opt for homemade or low-sugar versions of these condiments, or use vinegar, lemon juice, herbs, and spices to add flavor to your meals instead.

- **Sweetened Breakfast Cereals**: Breakfast cereals marketed to children are often high in added sugars and low in fiber, vitamins, and minerals. Starting your day with a bowl of sugary cereal can lead to blood sugar spikes and crashes, increasing the risk of fatty liver disease and other metabolic conditions. Choose whole grain cereals with little to no added sugars and top them with fresh fruit or nuts for added flavor and nutrition.

By limiting your intake of sugary foods and beverages like soda, candy, processed snacks, sweetened condiments, and sweetened breakfast cereals, you can reduce your risk of liver fat accumulation, insulin resistance, and complications associated with fatty liver disease. Instead, focus on whole, minimally processed foods and beverages to support liver health and overall well-being.

Processed Foods and Trans Fats

Processed foods are often high in unhealthy fats, added sugars, refined carbohydrates, and sodium, making them detrimental to liver health.

Trans fats, in particular, are highly inflammatory and can contribute to liver fat accumulation and insulin resistance. Avoiding processed foods and trans fats is essential for managing fatty liver disease and supporting liver health. Here are some processed foods and trans fats to avoid in your diet:

- **Packaged Snacks**: Packaged snacks like chips, crackers, pretzels, and snack cakes are often high in unhealthy fats, refined carbohydrates, and sodium. They're calorie-dense and nutrient-poor, and consuming them regularly can contribute to liver fat accumulation and inflammation. Choose healthier snack options like fresh fruit, nuts, seeds, or air-popped popcorn instead.

- **Frozen Meals**: Frozen meals like frozen dinners, pizzas, and entrees are convenient but often high in unhealthy fats, added sugars, and sodium. They're also typically low in fiber, vitamins, and minerals, making them a poor choice for individuals with fatty liver disease. Opt for homemade meals made with whole, minimally processed ingredients whenever possible to support liver health.

- **Packaged Baked Goods**: Packaged baked goods like cookies, cakes, muffins, and pastries are often high in unhealthy fats, refined carbohydrates, and added sugars. They're calorie-dense and nutrient-poor, and consuming them regularly can contribute to liver fat accumulation and insulin resistance. Limit your intake of packaged baked goods and opt for homemade versions made with healthier ingredients like whole grain flour, nuts, seeds, and fruit.

- **Margarine and Shortening**: Margarine and shortening are commonly used in baked goods, fried foods, and processed snacks as a replacement for butter. However, they're high in trans fats, which are highly inflammatory and can contribute to liver fat accumulation and insulin resistance. Avoid products containing margarine or shortening and opt for healthier fats like olive oil, avocado, nuts, and seeds instead.

- **Fast Food**: Fast food items like burgers, fries, chicken nuggets, and tacos are convenient but often high in unhealthy fats, refined carbohydrates, and sodium. They're also typically low in fiber, vitamins, and minerals, making them a poor choice for individuals with fatty liver disease. Limit your intake of fast food and opt for healthier options like homemade meals made with whole, minimally processed ingredients.

By avoiding processed foods and trans fats like packaged snacks, frozen meals, packaged baked goods, margarine, shortening, and fast food, you can reduce your risk of liver fat accumulation, inflammation, and complications associated with fatty liver disease. Instead, focus on whole, minimally processed foods made with healthy ingredients to support liver health and overall well-being.

Excessive Alcohol Consumption

Excessive alcohol consumption is a leading cause of fatty liver disease and can exacerbate liver inflammation, liver fat accumulation, and liver damage. Limiting or eliminating alcohol is essential for managing fatty liver disease and preventing further liver damage. Here are some reasons why excessive alcohol consumption should be avoided in individuals with fatty liver disease:

- **Liver Fat Accumulation**: Excessive alcohol consumption can lead to liver fat accumulation, a condition known as alcoholic fatty liver disease. Over time, this can progress to more severe forms of liver disease, including alcoholic hepatitis and cirrhosis. Limiting or eliminating alcohol is essential for reducing liver fat accumulation and preventing further liver damage.

- **Liver Inflammation**: Alcohol is a known liver toxin and can cause inflammation and damage to liver cells. Chronic inflammation of the liver can lead to liver fibrosis, scarring, and dysfunction. By avoiding excessive alcohol consumption, you can reduce inflammation and support liver health.

- **Liver Damage**: Long-term alcohol abuse can result in permanent liver damage and irreversible liver disease. Alcoholic liver disease is a leading cause of liver-related morbidity and mortality worldwide. By limiting or eliminating alcohol, you can reduce the risk of liver damage and improve liver function.

- **Risk of Complications**: Excessive alcohol consumption is associated with an increased risk of liver-related complications, including liver failure, liver cancer, and death. Individuals with fatty liver disease are already at an increased risk of these complications, and alcohol consumption further exacerbates the risk. By avoiding alcohol, you can reduce the risk of complications and improve overall health and well-being.

- **Interference with Treatment**: Excessive alcohol consumption can interfere with the effectiveness of treatment for fatty liver disease. Medications and lifestyle modifications may be less effective in individuals who continue to consume alcohol excessively. By abstaining from alcohol, you can optimize the effectiveness of treatment and support liver health.

BREAKFAST RECIPES

Avocado Toast with Poached Egg

Prep Time: 5 mins

Cook Time: 5 mins

Total Time: 10 mins

Servings: 2

Ingredients:

- 2 slices whole grain bread
- 1 ripe avocado
- 2 eggs
- Salt and pepper to taste
- Optional toppings: cherry tomatoes, microgreens, red pepper flakes

Directions:

1. Toast the whole grain bread until golden brown.
2. While the bread is toasting, poach the eggs in simmering water for about 3-4 minutes until the whites are set but the yolks are still runny.
3. Mash the ripe avocado in a bowl and season with salt and pepper to taste.
4. Spread the mashed avocado evenly onto the toasted bread slices.
5. Carefully place the poached eggs on top of the avocado spread.
6. Garnish with optional toppings like cherry tomatoes, microgreens, or red pepper flakes.

7. Serve immediately and enjoy!

Nutrition Facts (per serving):

- Calories: 250
- Total Fat: 15g
- Saturated Fat: 3g
- Cholesterol: 186mg
- Sodium: 258mg
- Total Carbohydrates: 20g
- Dietary Fiber: 9g
- Protein: 12g

Blueberry Chia Pudding

Prep Time: 5 mins

Chilling Time: 4 hours or overnight

Total Time: 4 hours 5 mins or overnight

Servings: 2

Ingredients:

- 1 cup unsweetened almond milk
- 1/4 cup chia seeds
- 1/2 teaspoon vanilla extract
- 1 tablespoon honey or maple syrup (optional)
- 1/2 cup fresh or frozen blueberries
- Optional toppings: sliced almonds, shredded coconut, additional blueberries

Directions:

1. In a mixing bowl, whisk together almond milk, chia seeds, vanilla extract, and honey or maple syrup (if using).

2. Let the mixture sit for 5 minutes, then whisk again to prevent clumping.

3. Gently stir in the blueberries.

4. Cover the bowl and refrigerate for at least 4 hours or overnight, until the chia pudding has thickened.

5. Once chilled and set, divide the chia pudding into serving bowls or glasses.

6. Top with optional toppings like sliced almonds, shredded coconut, or additional blueberries.

7. Serve chilled and enjoy!

Nutrition Facts (per serving):

- Calories: 190
- Total Fat: 9g
- Saturated Fat: 1g
- Cholesterol: 0mg
- Sodium: 90mg
- Total Carbohydrates: 23g
- Dietary Fiber: 11g
- Sugars: 7g
- Protein: 5g

Greek Yogurt Parfait

Prep Time: 5 mins

Total Time: 5 mins

Servings: 2

Ingredients:

- 1 cup plain Greek yogurt
- 1/2 cup granola (choose a low-sugar, whole grain variety)
- 1/2 cup mixed fresh berries (such as strawberries, blueberries, raspberries)
- 1 tablespoon honey or maple syrup (optional)
- Optional toppings: sliced almonds, shredded coconut, mint leaves

Directions:

1. In serving glasses or bowls, layer the Greek yogurt, granola, and mixed berries.
2. Drizzle with honey or maple syrup if desired.
3. Top with optional toppings like sliced almonds, shredded coconut, or mint leaves for garnish.
4. Serve immediately and enjoy!

Nutrition Facts (per serving):

- Calories: 250
- Total Fat: 6g
- Saturated Fat: 1g
- Cholesterol: 10mg
- Sodium: 80mg
- Total Carbohydrates: 37g
- Dietary Fiber: 5g

- Sugars: 18g

- Protein: 15g

Quinoa Breakfast Bowl

Prep Time: 5 mins

Cook Time: 15 mins

Total Time: 20 mins

Servings: 2

Ingredients:

- 1/2 cup quinoa

- 1 cup unsweetened almond milk

- 1 tablespoon honey or maple syrup

- 1/2 teaspoon ground cinnamon

- 1/4 teaspoon vanilla extract

- 1/2 cup mixed fresh berries (such as strawberries, blueberries, raspberries)

- 2 tablespoons chopped nuts (such as almonds, walnuts, pecans)

- Optional toppings: sliced banana, shredded coconut, chia seeds

Directions:

1. Rinse the quinoa under cold water, then combine it with almond milk in a saucepan.

2. Bring the mixture to a boil, then reduce the heat to low and simmer for 15 minutes, or until the quinoa is cooked and the liquid is absorbed.

3. Stir in honey or maple syrup, ground cinnamon, and vanilla extract.

4. Divide the cooked quinoa into serving bowls.

5. Top with mixed fresh berries and chopped nuts.

6. Garnish with optional toppings like sliced banana, shredded coconut, or chia seeds.

7. Serve warm and enjoy!

Nutrition Facts (per serving):

- Calories: 300

- Total Fat: 7g

- Saturated Fat: 1g

- Cholesterol: 0mg

- Sodium: 10mg

- Total Carbohydrates: 52g

- Dietary Fiber: 7g

- Sugars: 16g

- Protein: 9g

Egg and Vegetable Scramble

Prep Time: 10 mins

Cook Time: 10 mins

Total Time: 20 mins

Servings: 2

Ingredients:

- 4 large eggs

- 1/2 cup diced bell peppers (any color)

- 1/2 cup diced onions

- 1/2 cup chopped spinach

- 1 tablespoon olive oil

- Salt and pepper to taste
- Optional toppings: diced avocado, salsa, shredded cheese

Directions:

1. In a bowl, whisk together the eggs with salt and pepper until well combined.
2. Heat olive oil in a skillet over medium heat.
3. Add diced bell peppers and onions to the skillet and sauté until softened, about 3-4 minutes.
4. Add chopped spinach to the skillet and cook until wilted, about 1-2 minutes.
5. Pour the whisked eggs into the skillet and cook, stirring gently, until the eggs are scrambled and cooked through, about 3-4 minutes.
6. Divide the egg and vegetable scramble onto serving plates.
7. Garnish with optional toppings like diced avocado, salsa, or shredded cheese.
8. Serve hot and enjoy!

Nutrition Facts (per serving):

- Calories: 220
- Total Fat: 14g
- Saturated Fat: 3g
- Cholesterol: 372mg
- Sodium: 160mg
- Total Carbohydrates: 7g
- Dietary Fiber: 2g
- Sugars: 3g

- Protein: 16g

Quinoa Breakfast Bowl

Prep Time: 5 mins

Cook Time: 15 mins

Total Time: 20 mins

Servings: 2

Ingredients:

- 1/2 cup quinoa
- 1 cup unsweetened almond milk
- 1 tablespoon honey or maple syrup
- 1/2 teaspoon ground cinnamon
- 1/4 teaspoon vanilla extract
- 1/2 cup mixed fresh berries (such as strawberries, blueberries, raspberries)
- 2 tablespoons chopped nuts (such as almonds, walnuts, pecans)
- Optional toppings: sliced banana, shredded coconut, chia seeds

Directions:

1. Rinse the quinoa under cold water, then combine it with almond milk in a saucepan.
2. Bring the mixture to a boil, then reduce the heat to low and simmer for 15 minutes, or until the quinoa is cooked and the liquid is absorbed.
3. Stir in honey or maple syrup, ground cinnamon, and vanilla extract.
4. Divide the cooked quinoa into serving bowls.
5. Top with mixed fresh berries and chopped nuts.

6. Garnish with optional toppings like sliced banana, shredded coconut, or chia seeds.

7. Serve warm and enjoy!

Nutrition Facts (per serving):

- Calories: 300

- Total Fat: 7g

- Saturated Fat: 1g

- Cholesterol: 0mg

- Sodium: 10mg

- Total Carbohydrates: 52g

- Dietary Fiber: 7g

- Sugars: 16g

- Protein: 9g

Salmon and Avocado Breakfast Wrap

Prep Time: 10 mins

Cook Time: 5 mins

Total Time: 15 mins

Servings: 2

Ingredients:

- 2 whole grain or gluten-free tortillas

- 4 ounces cooked salmon (canned or fresh)

- 1 ripe avocado, sliced

- 1/4 cup diced tomatoes

- 2 tablespoons Greek yogurt

- 2 tablespoons chopped fresh cilantro

- Salt and pepper to taste

Directions:

1. Heat the tortillas in a skillet over medium heat until warm and pliable.
2. Place the warm tortillas on a flat surface.
3. Divide the cooked salmon evenly between the tortillas.
4. Top each tortilla with sliced avocado, diced tomatoes, Greek yogurt, and chopped cilantro.
5. Season with salt and pepper to taste.
6. Roll up the tortillas tightly to form wraps.
7. Slice the wraps in half diagonally and serve immediately.

Nutrition Facts (per serving):

- Calories: 320
- Total Fat: 15g
- Saturated Fat: 2g
- Cholesterol: 40mg
- Sodium: 310mg
- Total Carbohydrates: 28g
- Dietary Fiber: 6g
- Sugars: 2g
- Protein: 22g

Egg and Vegetable Frittata

Prep Time: 10 mins

Cook Time: 20 mins

Total Time: 30 mins

Servings: 4

Ingredients:

- 6 large eggs
- 1/4 cup unsweetened almond milk
- 1 cup chopped mixed vegetables (such as bell peppers, onions, spinach)
- 1/4 cup crumbled feta cheese
- 2 tablespoons chopped fresh herbs (such as parsley, chives, basil)
- Salt and pepper to taste
- Cooking spray or olive oil for greasing the pan

Directions:

1. Preheat the oven to 350°F (175°C).
2. In a mixing bowl, whisk together the eggs, almond milk, salt, and pepper until well combined.
3. Stir in the chopped mixed vegetables, crumbled feta cheese, and chopped fresh herbs.
4. Lightly grease a cast-iron skillet or oven-safe frying pan with cooking spray or olive oil.
5. Pour the egg and vegetable mixture into the greased skillet and spread it out evenly.
6. Transfer the skillet to the preheated oven and bake for 15-20 minutes, or until the frittata is set and lightly golden brown on top.

7. Remove the skillet from the oven and let the frittata cool for a
   few minutes before slicing and serving.

Nutrition Facts (per serving):

- Calories: 180
- Total Fat: 12g
- Saturated Fat: 4g
- Cholesterol: 280mg
- Sodium: 320mg
- Total Carbohydrates: 6g
- Dietary Fiber: 2g
- Sugars: 2g
- Protein: 13g

Spinach and Mushroom Omelette

Prep Time: 5 mins

Cook Time: 10 mins

Total Time: 15 mins

Servings: 2

Ingredients:

- 4 large eggs
- 2 tablespoons unsweetened almond milk
- 1 cup fresh spinach leaves
- 1/2 cup sliced mushrooms
- 1/4 cup diced onions
- 1/4 cup shredded mozzarella cheese
- Salt and pepper to taste

- Cooking spray or olive oil for greasing the pan

Directions:

1. In a mixing bowl, whisk together the eggs, almond milk, salt, and pepper until well combined.
2. Heat a non-stick skillet over medium heat and lightly grease it with cooking spray or olive oil.
3. Add the diced onions and sliced mushrooms to the skillet and sauté until softened, about 3-4 minutes.
4. Add the fresh spinach leaves to the skillet and cook until wilted, about 1-2 minutes.
5. Pour the whisked egg mixture into the skillet, covering the sautéed vegetables evenly.
6. Cook the omelette for 3-4 minutes, or until the edges begin to set.
7. Sprinkle the shredded mozzarella cheese over one half of the omelette.
8. Carefully fold the other half of the omelette over the cheese to form a half-moon shape.
9. Cook for an additional 2-3 minutes, or until the cheese is melted and the omelette is cooked through.
10. Slide the omelette onto a serving plate, slice it in half, and serve immediately.

Nutrition Facts (per serving):

- Calories: 220
- Total Fat: 15g
- Saturated Fat: 5g

- Cholesterol: 370mg

- Sodium: 270mg

- Total Carbohydrates: 5g

- Dietary Fiber: 2g

- Sugars: 2g

- Protein: 17g

Chia Seed Breakfast Pudding

Prep Time: 5 mins

Chilling Time: 4 hours or overnight

Total Time: 4 hours 5 mins or overnight

Servings: 2

Ingredients:

- 1/4 cup chia seeds

- 1 cup unsweetened almond milk

- 1 tablespoon honey or maple syrup (optional)

- 1/2 teaspoon vanilla extract

- 1/2 cup mixed fresh berries (such as strawberries, blueberries, raspberries)

- 2 tablespoons chopped nuts (such as almonds, walnuts, pecans)

- Optional toppings: sliced banana, shredded coconut, hemp seeds

Directions:

1. In a mixing bowl, whisk together chia seeds, almond milk, honey or maple syrup (if using), and vanilla extract until well combined.

2. Let the mixture sit for 5 minutes, then whisk again to prevent clumping.

3. Cover the bowl and refrigerate for at least 4 hours or overnight, until the chia pudding has thickened.

4. Once chilled and set, divide the chia pudding into serving bowls.

5. Top with mixed fresh berries and chopped nuts.

6. Garnish with optional toppings like sliced banana, shredded coconut, or hemp seeds.

7. Serve chilled and enjoy!

Nutrition Facts (per serving):

- Calories: 230
- Total Fat: 13g
- Saturated Fat: 1g
- Cholesterol: 0mg
- Sodium: 80mg
- Total Carbohydrates: 27g
- Dietary Fiber: 11g
- Sugars: 12g
- Protein: 6g

Turkey and Vegetable Breakfast Skillet

Prep Time: 10 mins

Cook Time: 15 mins

Total Time: 25 mins

Servings: 2

Ingredients:

- 4 large eggs
- 4 ounces lean turkey sausage, sliced
- 1 cup diced bell peppers (any color)
- 1/2 cup diced onions
- 1 cup chopped spinach
- Salt and pepper to taste
- Cooking spray or olive oil for greasing the skillet

Directions:

1. In a mixing bowl, whisk together the eggs with salt and pepper until well combined.
2. Heat a non-stick skillet over medium heat and lightly grease it with cooking spray or olive oil.
3. Add the sliced turkey sausage to the skillet and cook until browned and cooked through, about 5-6 minutes.
4. Add the diced bell peppers and onions to the skillet and sauté until softened, about 3-4 minutes.
5. Stir in the chopped spinach and cook until wilted, about 1-2 minutes.
6. Pour the whisked eggs into the skillet, covering the sausage and vegetables evenly.
7. Cook the mixture, stirring gently, until the eggs are scrambled and cooked through, about 3-4 minutes.
8. Divide the turkey and vegetable breakfast skillet onto serving plates.
9. Serve hot and enjoy!

Nutrition Facts (per serving):

- Calories: 280
- Total Fat: 15g
- Saturated Fat: 4g
- Cholesterol: 380mg
- Sodium: 570mg
- Total Carbohydrates: 11g
- Dietary Fiber: 3g
- Sugars: 5g
- Protein: 23g

Spinach and Mushroom Breakfast Wrap

Prep Time: 10 mins

Cook Time: 10 mins

Total Time: 20 mins

Servings: 2

Ingredients:

- 2 whole grain or gluten-free tortillas
- 1 cup chopped spinach
- 1/2 cup sliced mushrooms
- 1/4 cup diced onions
- 2 large eggs
- 1/4 cup shredded mozzarella cheese
- Salt and pepper to taste
- Cooking spray or olive oil for greasing the skillet

Directions:

1. Heat a non-stick skillet over medium heat and lightly grease it with cooking spray or olive oil.
2. Add the chopped spinach, sliced mushrooms, and diced onions to the skillet and sauté until softened, about 3-4 minutes.
3. In a separate bowl, whisk together the eggs with salt and pepper until well combined.
4. Pour the whisked eggs into the skillet, covering the sautéed vegetables evenly.
5. Cook the mixture, stirring gently, until the eggs are scrambled and cooked through, about 3-4 minutes.
6. Place a tortilla on a flat surface and sprinkle half of the shredded mozzarella cheese evenly over the tortilla.
7. Spoon half of the cooked egg and vegetable mixture onto the tortilla.
8. Roll up the tortilla tightly to form a wrap.
9. Repeat the process with the remaining tortilla and ingredients.
10. Slice the wraps in half diagonally and serve immediately.

Nutrition Facts (per serving):

- Calories: 250
- Total Fat: 10g
- Saturated Fat: 4g
- Cholesterol: 195mg
- Sodium: 380mg
- Total Carbohydrates: 22g
- Dietary Fiber: 5g
- Sugars: 3g

- Protein: 16g

Berry and Greek Yogurt Parfait

Prep Time: 5 mins

Total Time: 5 mins

Servings: 2

Ingredients:

- 1 cup plain Greek yogurt
- 1/2 cup mixed fresh berries (such as strawberries, blueberries, raspberries)
- 1/4 cup granola (choose a low-sugar, whole grain variety)
- 1 tablespoon honey or maple syrup (optional)
- Optional toppings: sliced almonds, shredded coconut, chia seeds

Directions:

1. In serving glasses or bowls, layer the Greek yogurt, mixed fresh berries, and granola.
2. Drizzle with honey or maple syrup if desired.
3. Top with optional toppings like sliced almonds, shredded coconut, or chia seeds.
4. Serve immediately and enjoy!

Nutrition Facts (per serving):

- Calories: 220
- Total Fat: 5g
- Saturated Fat: 1g
- Cholesterol: 10mg
- Sodium: 70mg

- Total Carbohydrates: 30g

- Dietary Fiber: 3g

- Sugars: 20g

- Protein: 15g

Egg and Spinach Breakfast Muffins

Prep Time: 10 mins

Cook Time: 20 mins

Total Time: 30 mins

Servings: 6 muffins

Ingredients:

- 6 large eggs

- 1 cup fresh spinach, chopped

- 1/2 cup diced bell peppers (any color)

- 1/4 cup diced onions

- 1/4 cup shredded mozzarella cheese

- Salt and pepper to taste

- Cooking spray or olive oil for greasing the muffin tin

Directions:

1. Preheat the oven to 350°F (175°C) and grease a muffin tin with cooking spray or olive oil.

2. In a mixing bowl, whisk together the eggs with salt and pepper until well combined.

3. Stir in the chopped spinach, diced bell peppers, diced onions, and shredded mozzarella cheese until evenly distributed.

4. Pour the egg mixture into the greased muffin tin, filling each cup about 3/4 full.

5. Bake in the preheated oven for 18-20 minutes, or until the egg muffins are set and lightly golden brown on top.

6. Remove the muffin tin from the oven and let the egg muffins cool for a few minutes before removing them from the tin.

7. Serve warm or at room temperature and enjoy!

Nutrition Facts (per serving - 1 muffin):

- Calories: 90
- Total Fat: 6g
- Saturated Fat: 2g
- Cholesterol: 190mg
- Sodium: 120mg
- Total Carbohydrates: 2g
- Dietary Fiber: 1g
- Sugars: 1g
- Protein: 8g

Green Smoothie Bowl

Prep Time: 5 mins

Total Time: 5 mins

Servings: 1 bowl

Ingredients:

- 1 cup fresh spinach leaves
- 1/2 frozen banana
- 1/2 cup frozen pineapple chunks
- 1/2 cup unsweetened almond milk
- 1 tablespoon almond butter

- Optional toppings: sliced banana, fresh berries, shredded coconut, chia seeds

Directions:

1. In a blender, combine the fresh spinach leaves, frozen banana, frozen pineapple chunks, almond milk, and almond butter.
2. Blend until smooth and creamy, adding more almond milk if needed to reach your desired consistency.
3. Pour the smoothie into a bowl and top with optional toppings like sliced banana, fresh berries, shredded coconut, or chia seeds.
4. Serve immediately and enjoy!

Nutrition Facts (per serving):

- Calories: 250
- Total Fat: 11g
- Saturated Fat: 1g
- Cholesterol: 0mg
- Sodium: 160mg
- Total Carbohydrates: 34g
- Dietary Fiber: 7g
- Sugars: 20g
- Protein: 6g

Smoked Salmon Breakfast Wrap

Prep Time: 10 mins

Cook Time: 5 mins

Total Time: 15 mins

Servings: 2 wraps

Ingredients:

- 2 whole grain or gluten-free tortillas
- 4 ounces smoked salmon
- 1/4 cup Greek yogurt
- 2 tablespoons capers
- 1/4 cup sliced cucumbers
- 1/4 cup shredded carrots
- 1 tablespoon chopped fresh dill
- Salt and pepper to taste

Directions:

1. Lay the tortillas flat on a clean surface.
2. Spread Greek yogurt evenly over each tortilla.
3. Divide the smoked salmon, capers, sliced cucumbers, shredded carrots, and chopped fresh dill between the tortillas.
4. Season with salt and pepper to taste.
5. Roll up the tortillas tightly to form wraps.
6. Slice the wraps in half diagonally and serve immediately.

Nutrition Facts (per serving - 1 wrap):

- Calories: 210
- Total Fat: 8g
- Saturated Fat: 1g
- Cholesterol: 15mg
- Sodium: 550mg
- Total Carbohydrates: 22g

- Dietary Fiber: 3g

- Sugars: 2g

- Protein: 16g

LUNCH RECIPES

Quinoa Salad with Grilled Chicken

Prep Time: 10 mins

Cook Time: 20 mins

Total Time: 30 mins

Servings: 2

Ingredients:

- 1/2 cup quinoa
- 1 cup water or low-sodium chicken broth
- 2 boneless, skinless chicken breasts
- 1 tablespoon olive oil
- Salt and pepper to taste
- 2 cups mixed salad greens (such as spinach, arugula, kale)
- 1/2 cup cherry tomatoes, halved
- 1/4 cup diced cucumber
- 1/4 cup diced red onion
- 2 tablespoons crumbled feta cheese
- 2 tablespoons balsamic vinaigrette

Directions:

1. Rinse the quinoa under cold water and drain.
2. In a saucepan, bring the water or chicken broth to a boil. Add the quinoa, reduce heat to low, cover, and simmer for 15-20 minutes, or until the quinoa is tender and the liquid is absorbed. Remove from heat and let it cool.

3. Preheat the grill or grill pan over medium-high heat. Season the chicken breasts with olive oil, salt, and pepper.

4. Grill the chicken breasts for 6-8 minutes on each side, or until cooked through and no longer pink in the center. Remove from heat and let them rest for a few minutes before slicing.

5. In a large mixing bowl, combine the cooked quinoa, mixed salad greens, cherry tomatoes, diced cucumber, and diced red onion.

6. Top the salad with sliced grilled chicken and crumbled feta cheese.

7. Drizzle with balsamic vinaigrette and toss gently to combine.

8. Divide the quinoa salad onto serving plates and serve immediately.

Nutrition Facts (per serving):

- Calories: 380
- Total Fat: 15g
- Saturated Fat: 3g
- Cholesterol: 80mg
- Sodium: 320mg
- Total Carbohydrates: 32g
- Dietary Fiber: 5g
- Sugars: 4g
- Protein: 30g

Salmon and Vegetable Stir-Fry

Prep Time: 15 mins

Cook Time: 10 mins

Total Time: 25 mins

Servings: 2

Ingredients:

- 2 salmon fillets
- 2 tablespoons low-sodium soy sauce
- 1 tablespoon rice vinegar
- 1 tablespoon honey or maple syrup
- 1 tablespoon sesame oil
- 2 cloves garlic, minced
- 1 teaspoon minced ginger
- 2 cups mixed stir-fry vegetables (such as bell peppers, broccoli, snap peas)
- 2 cups cooked brown rice
- 1 tablespoon chopped green onions (for garnish)
- Sesame seeds (for garnish)

Directions:

1. In a small bowl, whisk together soy sauce, rice vinegar, honey or maple syrup, sesame oil, minced garlic, and minced ginger to make the sauce.

2. Heat a non-stick skillet or wok over medium-high heat. Add the salmon fillets and cook for 3-4 minutes on each side, or until cooked through. Remove from heat and set aside.

3. In the same skillet or wok, add the mixed stir-fry vegetables and cook for 3-4 minutes, or until crisp-tender.

4. Pour the prepared sauce over the vegetables and stir to coat evenly. Cook for an additional 1-2 minutes, or until the sauce thickens slightly.

5. Serve the stir-fry vegetables over cooked brown rice, topped with cooked salmon fillets.

6. Garnish with chopped green onions and sesame seeds.

7. Serve hot and enjoy!

Nutrition Facts (per serving):

- Calories: 420
- Total Fat: 15g
- Saturated Fat: 3g
- Cholesterol: 60mg
- Sodium: 500mg
- Total Carbohydrates: 48g
- Dietary Fiber: 6g
- Sugars: 9g
- Protein: 26g

Turkey and Quinoa Stuffed Bell Peppers

Prep Time: 15 mins

Cook Time: 45 mins

Total Time: 1 hour

Servings: 2

Ingredients:

- 2 large bell peppers (any color), halved and seeded
- 1/2 cup quinoa

- 1 cup low-sodium chicken broth
- 8 ounces lean ground turkey
- 1/2 cup diced tomatoes
- 1/4 cup diced onions
- 1/4 cup diced zucchini
- 1/4 cup shredded mozzarella cheese
- 1 teaspoon dried Italian seasoning
- Salt and pepper to taste

Directions:

1. Preheat the oven to 375°F (190°C) and lightly grease a baking dish.
2. Place the halved bell peppers in the prepared baking dish, cut side up.
3. In a saucepan, bring the chicken broth to a boil. Add the quinoa, reduce heat to low, cover, and simmer for 15-20 minutes, or until the quinoa is tender and the liquid is absorbed. Remove from heat and let it cool.
4. In a skillet, cook the ground turkey over medium heat until browned and cooked through. Drain any excess fat.
5. Add the diced tomatoes, onions, zucchini, cooked quinoa, dried Italian seasoning, salt, and pepper to the skillet with the cooked turkey. Stir to combine.
6. Spoon the turkey and quinoa mixture into the halved bell peppers, dividing it evenly.
7. Top each stuffed pepper with shredded mozzarella cheese.

8. Cover the baking dish with aluminum foil and bake in the preheated oven for 25-30 minutes, or until the peppers are tender and the cheese is melted and bubbly.

9. Remove from the oven and let the stuffed peppers cool for a few minutes before serving.

Nutrition Facts (per serving):

- Calories: 340
- Total Fat: 10g
- Saturated Fat: 3g
- Cholesterol: 65mg
- Sodium: 420mg
- Total Carbohydrates: 32g
- Dietary Fiber: 5g
- Sugars: 6g
- Protein: 30g

Mediterranean Chickpea Salad

Prep Time: 15 mins

Cook Time: 0 mins

Total Time: 15 mins

Servings: 2

Ingredients:

- 1 can (15 ounces) chickpeas, drained and rinsed
- 1 cup cherry tomatoes, halved
- 1/2 cup diced cucumber
- 1/4 cup diced red onion

- 1/4 cup chopped fresh parsley

- 2 tablespoons crumbled feta cheese

- 2 tablespoons extra virgin olive oil

- 1 tablespoon lemon juice

- 1 teaspoon dried oregano

- Salt and pepper to taste

Directions:

1. In a large mixing bowl, combine the chickpeas, cherry tomatoes, diced cucumber, diced red onion, chopped fresh parsley, and crumbled feta cheese.

2. In a small bowl, whisk together the extra virgin olive oil, lemon juice, dried oregano, salt, and pepper to make the dressing.

3. Pour the dressing over the chickpea salad and toss gently to coat evenly.

4. Serve the Mediterranean chickpea salad chilled or at room temperature.

Nutrition Facts (per serving):

- Calories: 320

- Total Fat: 16g

- Saturated Fat: 3g

- Cholesterol: 5mg

- Sodium: 330mg

- Total Carbohydrates: 37g

- Dietary Fiber: 9g

- Sugars: 6g

- Protein: 10g

Turkey and Vegetable Stir-Fry

Prep Time: 15 mins

Cook Time: 10 mins

Total Time: 25 mins

Servings: 2

Ingredients:

- 2 turkey breasts, sliced thinly
- 2 cups mixed vegetables (bell peppers, broccoli, snap peas)
- 2 tablespoons low-sodium soy sauce
- 1 tablespoon sesame oil
- 1 tablespoon honey or maple syrup
- 1 teaspoon minced garlic
- 1 teaspoon minced ginger
- 2 cups cooked brown rice
- Salt and pepper to taste
- Optional garnish: sliced green onions, sesame seeds

Directions:

1. In a small bowl, mix soy sauce, sesame oil, honey or maple syrup, minced garlic, and minced ginger to make the sauce.

2. Heat a non-stick skillet over medium-high heat. Add sliced turkey breasts and cook until browned and cooked through, about 5-6 minutes. Remove from skillet and set aside.

3. In the same skillet, add mixed vegetables and stir-fry until tender-crisp, about 3-4 minutes.

4. Return cooked turkey to the skillet. Pour the sauce over the turkey and vegetables. Stir until everything is evenly coated and heated through.

5. Serve turkey and vegetable stir-fry over cooked brown rice. Garnish with sliced green onions and sesame seeds if desired.

6. Season with salt and pepper to taste.

7. Serve hot and enjoy!

Nutrition Facts (per serving):

- Calories: 380
- Total Fat: 8g
- Saturated Fat: 1.5g
- Cholesterol: 60mg
- Sodium: 580mg
- Total Carbohydrates: 52g
- Dietary Fiber: 6g
- Sugars: 8g
- Protein: 28g

Baked Salmon with Roasted Vegetables

Prep Time: 15 mins

Cook Time: 25 mins

Total Time: 40 mins

Servings: 2

Ingredients:

- 2 salmon fillets

- 2 cups mixed vegetables (zucchini, cherry tomatoes, bell peppers)
- 2 tablespoons olive oil
- 1 teaspoon dried Italian herbs
- Salt and pepper to taste
- Lemon wedges (for serving)

Directions:

1. Preheat the oven to 400°F (200°C). Line a baking sheet with parchment paper.
2. Place salmon fillets and mixed vegetables on the prepared baking sheet.
3. Drizzle olive oil over salmon and vegetables. Sprinkle with dried Italian herbs, salt, and pepper.
4. Bake in the preheated oven for 20-25 minutes, or until salmon is cooked through and vegetables are tender.
5. Remove from the oven and let it rest for a few minutes before serving.
6. Serve baked salmon and roasted vegetables with lemon wedges on the side.
7. Enjoy your nutritious meal!

Nutrition Facts (per serving):

- Calories: 350
- Total Fat: 20g
- Saturated Fat: 3g
- Cholesterol: 60mg
- Sodium: 180mg

- Total Carbohydrates: 15g

- Dietary Fiber: 5g

- Sugars: 7g

- Protein: 30g

Quinoa and Black Bean Salad

Prep Time: 15 mins

Cook Time: 15 mins

Total Time: 30 mins

Servings: 2

Ingredients:

- 1/2 cup quinoa

- 1 cup water or low-sodium vegetable broth

- 1 can (15 ounces) black beans, drained and rinsed

- 1 cup cherry tomatoes, halved

- 1/2 cup diced bell peppers (any color)

- 1/4 cup diced red onions

- 1/4 cup chopped cilantro

- 2 tablespoons lime juice

- 2 tablespoons olive oil

- 1 teaspoon ground cumin

- Salt and pepper to taste

- Optional garnish: avocado slices, sliced jalapenos

Directions:

1. Rinse quinoa under cold water and drain.

2. In a saucepan, bring water or vegetable broth to a boil. Add quinoa, reduce heat to low, cover, and simmer for 15 minutes,

or until quinoa is tender and liquid is absorbed. Remove from heat and let it cool.

3. In a large mixing bowl, combine cooked quinoa, black beans, cherry tomatoes, diced bell peppers, diced red onions, and chopped cilantro.

4. In a small bowl, whisk together lime juice, olive oil, ground cumin, salt, and pepper to make the dressing.

5. Pour the dressing over the quinoa salad and toss gently to combine.

6. Serve quinoa and black bean salad chilled or at room temperature.

7. Garnish with avocado slices and sliced jalapenos if desired.

8. Enjoy your healthy and flavorful lunch!

Nutrition Facts (per serving):

- Calories: 320
- Total Fat: 12g
- Saturated Fat: 2g
- Cholesterol: 0mg
- Sodium: 380m
- Total Carbohydrates: 45g
- Dietary Fiber: 10g
- Sugars: 5g
- Protein: 12g

Grilled Chicken Caesar Salad

Prep Time: 15 mins

Cook Time: 10 mins

Total Time: 25 mins

Servings: 2

Ingredients:

- 2 boneless, skinless chicken breasts
- 4 cups chopped romaine lettuce
- 1/4 cup grated Parmesan cheese
- 1/2 cup croutons
- 2 tablespoons Caesar dressing (store-bought or homemade)
- Salt and pepper to taste
- Lemon wedges (for serving)

Directions:

1. Preheat the grill or grill pan over medium-high heat.
2. Season chicken breasts with salt and pepper.
3. Grill chicken breasts for 5-6 minutes on each side, or until cooked through and no longer pink in the center. Remove from heat and let them rest for a few minutes before slicing.
4. In a large mixing bowl, combine chopped romaine lettuce, grated Parmesan cheese, and croutons.
5. Add sliced grilled chicken on top of the salad.
6. Drizzle Caesar dressing over the salad and toss gently to coat evenly.
7. Serve grilled chicken Caesar salad with lemon wedges on the side.
8. Enjoy this classic and satisfying salad!

Nutrition Facts (per serving):

- Calories: 300
- Total Fat: 12g
- Saturated Fat: 3g
- Cholesterol: 80mg
- Sodium: 580mg
- Total Carbohydrates: 14g
- Dietary Fiber: 3g
- Sugars: 2g
- Protein: 35g

Grilled Lemon Herb Chicken with Steamed Vegetables

Prep Time: 10 mins

Cook Time: 15 mins

Total Time: 25 mins

Servings: 2

Ingredients:

- 2 boneless, skinless chicken breasts
- 1 lemon, juiced and zested
- 2 cloves garlic, minced
- 1 tablespoon chopped fresh parsley
- 1 tablespoon chopped fresh thyme
- Salt and pepper to taste
- 2 cups mixed vegetables (broccoli, carrots, cauliflower)
- Cooking spray or olive oil for greasing

Directions:

1. In a small bowl, whisk together lemon juice, lemon zest, minced garlic, chopped parsley, chopped thyme, salt, and pepper to make the marinade.
2. Place chicken breasts in a shallow dish and pour the marinade over them. Turn to coat evenly. Let marinate for at least 30 minutes in the refrigerator.
3. Preheat grill or grill pan over medium-high heat. Grease with cooking spray or olive oil.
4. Remove chicken breasts from marinade and discard excess marinade. Grill chicken for 6-7 minutes on each side, or until cooked through and no longer pink in the center.
5. While chicken is grilling, steam mixed vegetables until tender, about 5-7 minutes.
6. Serve grilled lemon herb chicken with steamed vegetables.
7. Enjoy your nutritious and flavorful meal!

Nutrition Facts (per serving):

- Calories: 250
- Total Fat: 5g
- Saturated Fat: 1g
- Cholesterol: 90mg
- Sodium: 120mg
- Total Carbohydrates: 10g
- Dietary Fiber: 4g
- Sugars: 3g
- Protein: 40g

Vegetarian Quinoa Buddha Bowl

Prep Time: 15 mins

Cook Time: 20 mins

Total Time: 35 mins

Servings: 2

Ingredients:

- 1/2 cup quinoa
- 1 cup water or vegetable broth
- 1 cup cooked chickpeas
- 1 cup mixed greens (spinach, kale, arugula)
- 1/2 cup cherry tomatoes, halved
- 1/2 avocado, sliced
- 1/4 cup shredded carrots
- 1/4 cup shredded red cabbage
- 2 tablespoons hummus
- 2 tablespoons balsamic vinaigrette
- Salt and pepper to taste

Directions:

1. Rinse quinoa under cold water and drain. In a saucepan, bring water or vegetable broth to a boil. Add quinoa, reduce heat to low, cover, and simmer for 15 minutes, or until quinoa is tender and liquid is absorbed. Remove from heat and let it cool.

2. In a serving bowl, arrange cooked quinoa, cooked chickpeas, mixed greens, cherry tomatoes, avocado slices, shredded carrots, and shredded red cabbage.

3. Drizzle with hummus and balsamic vinaigrette. Season with salt and pepper to taste.

4. Serve vegetarian quinoa Buddha bowl immediately.

5. Enjoy this colorful and nutrient-rich meal!

Nutrition Facts (per serving):

- Calories: 380
- Total Fat: 15g
- Saturated Fat: 2g
- Cholesterol: 0mg
- Sodium: 250mg
- Total Carbohydrates: 50g
- Dietary Fiber: 12g
- Sugars: 6g
- Protein: 15g

Salmon and Asparagus Foil Packets

Prep Time: 10 mins

Cook Time: 20 mins

Total Time: 30 mins

Servings: 2

Ingredients:

- 2 salmon fillets
- 1 bunch asparagus, trimmed
- 1 lemon, thinly sliced
- 2 cloves garlic, minced
- 2 tablespoons olive oil

- Salt and pepper to taste
- Fresh dill (optional, for garnish)

Directions:

1. Preheat oven to 400°F (200°C).
2. Cut two sheets of aluminum foil, large enough to wrap each salmon fillet and asparagus.
3. Place one salmon fillet in the center of each foil sheet. Arrange asparagus spears around salmon.
4. Top each salmon fillet with minced garlic and lemon slices. Drizzle with olive oil. Season with salt and pepper.
5. Fold up the sides of the foil to create a packet, sealing tightly.
6. Place foil packets on a baking sheet and bake in preheated oven for 15-20 minutes, or until salmon is cooked through and asparagus is tender.
7. Carefully open foil packets, garnish with fresh dill if desired, and serve immediately.
8. Enjoy this simple and delicious meal!

Nutrition Facts (per serving):

- Calories: 320
- Total Fat: 18g
- Saturated Fat: 3g
- Cholesterol: 80mg
- Sodium: 160mg
- Total Carbohydrates: 7g
- Dietary Fiber: 3g
- Sugars: 2g

- Protein: 34g

Greek Turkey Meatball Lettuce Wraps

Prep Time: 15 mins

Cook Time: 15 mins

Total Time: 30 mins

Servings: 2

Ingredients:

- 1/2 lb ground turkey
- 1/4 cup whole wheat breadcrumbs
- 1/4 cup crumbled feta cheese
- 2 tablespoons chopped fresh parsley
- 1 teaspoon dried oregano
- 1/2 teaspoon garlic powder
- Salt and pepper to taste
- 4 large lettuce leaves (such as romaine or butter lettuce)
- Tzatziki sauce (store-bought or homemade, for serving)
- Diced tomatoes, cucumber, red onion (optional, for serving)

Directions:

1. Preheat oven to 400°F (200°C). Line a baking sheet with parchment paper.
2. In a mixing bowl, combine ground turkey, breadcrumbs, feta cheese, chopped parsley, dried oregano, garlic powder, salt, and pepper. Mix until well combined.
3. Shape the turkey mixture into small meatballs, about 1-inch in diameter, and place them on the prepared baking sheet.

4. Bake in preheated oven for 12-15 minutes, or until meatballs are cooked through and lightly browned.

5. To assemble the lettuce wraps, place 2 lettuce leaves on each plate. Divide cooked turkey meatballs evenly among the lettuce leaves.

6. Drizzle with tzatziki sauce and top with diced tomatoes, cucumber, and red onion if desired.

7. Serve Greek turkey meatball lettuce wraps immediately.

8. Enjoy this light and flavorful lunch option!

Nutrition Facts (per serving):

- Calories: 280
- Total Fat: 14g
- Saturated Fat: 4g
- Cholesterol: 80mg
- Sodium: 350mg
- Total Carbohydrates: 9g
- Dietary Fiber: 2g
- Sugars: 2g
- Protein: 29g

Tuna and White Bean Salad

Prep Time: 10 mins

Cook Time: 0 mins

Total Time: 10 mins

Servings: 2

Ingredients:

- 1 can (5 oz) tuna, drained
- 1 can (15 oz.) white beans, drained and rinsed
- 1/4 cup diced red onion
- 1/4 cup chopped celery
- 1 tablespoon chopped fresh parsley
- 1 tablespoon lemon juice
- 1 tablespoon olive oil
- Salt and pepper to taste
- Mixed greens or lettuce leaves (for serving)

Directions:

1. In a large mixing bowl, combine drained tuna, white beans, diced red onion, chopped celery, and chopped parsley.
2. Drizzle with lemon juice and olive oil. Season with salt and pepper to taste.
3. Toss until well combined.
4. Serve tuna and white bean salad over mixed greens or lettuce leaves.
5. Enjoy this protein-packed salad for a satisfying lunch!

Nutrition Facts (per serving):

- Calories: 280
- Total Fat: 9g
- Saturated Fat: 1g
- Cholesterol: 15mg
- Sodium: 490mg
- Total Carbohydrates: 28g
- Dietary Fiber: 7g

- Sugars: 1g

- Protein: 25g

Mediterranean Quinoa Salad

Prep Time: 15 mins

Cook Time: 15 mins

Total Time: 30 mins

Servings: 2

Ingredients:

- 1/2 cup quinoa

- 1 cup water or low-sodium vegetable broth

- 1/4 cup diced cucumber

- 1/4 cup diced tomatoes

- 1/4 cup diced red bell pepper

- 1/4 cup chopped Kalamata olives

- 2 tablespoons crumbled feta cheese

- 2 tablespoons chopped fresh parsley

- 2 tablespoons lemon juice

- 1 tablespoon olive oil

- Salt and pepper to taste

Directions:

1. Rinse quinoa under cold water and drain.

2. In a saucepan, bring water or vegetable broth to a boil. Add quinoa, reduce heat to low, cover, and simmer for 15 minutes, or until quinoa is tender and liquid is absorbed. Remove from heat and let it cool.

3. In a large mixing bowl, combine cooked quinoa, diced cucumber, diced tomatoes, diced red bell pepper, chopped Kalamata olives, crumbled feta cheese, and chopped parsley.

4. In a small bowl, whisk together lemon juice, olive oil, salt, and pepper to make the dressing.

5. Pour the dressing over the quinoa salad and toss gently to coat evenly.

6. Serve Mediterranean quinoa salad chilled or at room temperature.

7. Enjoy this refreshing and nutritious salad!

Nutrition Facts (per serving):

- Calories: 320
- Total Fat: 14g
- Saturated Fat: 3g
- Cholesterol: 8mg
- Sodium: 480m
- Total Carbohydrates: 39g
- Dietary Fiber: 6g
- Sugars: 3g
- Protein: 10g

Chicken and Vegetable Stir-Fry

Prep Time: 15 mins

Cook Time: 10 mins

Total Time: 25 mins

Servings: 2

Ingredients:

- 2 boneless, skinless chicken breasts, sliced thinly
- 2 cups mixed vegetables (bell peppers, broccoli, snap peas)
- 2 tablespoons low-sodium soy sauce
- 1 tablespoon sesame oil
- 1 tablespoon honey or maple syrup
- 1 teaspoon minced garlic
- 1 teaspoon minced ginger
- 2 cups cooked brown rice
- Salt and pepper to taste
- Optional garnish: sliced green onions, sesame seeds

Directions:

1. In a small bowl, mix soy sauce, sesame oil, honey or maple syrup, minced garlic, and minced ginger to make the sauce.

2. Heat a non-stick skillet over medium-high heat. Add sliced chicken breasts and cook until browned and cooked through, about 5-6 minutes. Remove from skillet and set aside.

3. In the same skillet, add mixed vegetables and stir-fry until tender-crisp, about 3-4 minutes.

4. Return cooked chicken to the skillet. Pour the sauce over the chicken and vegetables. Stir until everything is evenly coated and heated through.

5. Serve chicken and vegetable stir-fry over cooked brown rice. Garnish with sliced green onions and sesame seeds if desired.

6. Season with salt and pepper to taste.

7. Serve hot and enjoy!

Nutrition Facts (per serving):

- Calories: 380
- Total Fat: 8g
- Saturated Fat: 1.5g
- Cholesterol: 60mg
- Sodium: 580mg
- Total Carbohydrates: 52g
- Dietary Fiber: 6g
- Sugars: 8g
- Protein: 28g

Salmon and Avocado Wrap

Prep Time: 10 mins

Cook Time: 10 mins

Total Time: 20 mins

Servings: 2

Ingredients:

- 2 salmon fillets
- 2 whole grain tortillas or wraps
- 1 ripe avocado, sliced
- 1 cup shredded lettuce
- 1/4 cup diced tomatoes
- 2 tablespoons Greek yogurt or sour cream
- 1 tablespoon lime juice
- Salt and pepper to taste

Directions:

1. Season salmon fillets with salt and pepper. Grill or pan-sear salmon until cooked through, about 4-5 minutes per side.
2. In a small bowl, mix Greek yogurt or sour cream with lime juice to make the dressing.
3. Warm tortillas or wraps according to package instructions.
4. Place a salmon fillet in the center of each tortilla or wrap. Top with sliced avocado, shredded lettuce, diced tomatoes, and drizzle with the lime yogurt dressing.
5. Fold in the sides of the tortillas or wraps and roll tightly.
6. Serve salmon and avocado wraps immediately.
7. Enjoy this delicious and satisfying lunch option!

Nutrition Facts (per serving):
- Calories: 340
- Total Fat: 17g
- Saturated Fat: 3g
- Cholesterol: 70mg
- Sodium: 280mg
- Total Carbohydrates: 22g
- Dietary Fiber: 6g
- Sugars: 2g
- Protein: 26g

DINNER RECIPES

Baked Lemon Herb Salmon

Prep Time: 10 mins

Cook Time: 15 mins

Total Time: 25 mins

Servings: 2

Ingredients:

- 2 salmon fillets
- 1 lemon, thinly sliced
- 2 cloves garlic, minced
- 1 tablespoon chopped fresh parsley
- 1 tablespoon chopped fresh dill
- 1 tablespoon olive oil
- Salt and pepper to taste
- Optional: lemon wedges for serving

Directions:

1. Preheat oven to 400°F (200°C). Line a baking sheet with parchment paper.
2. Place salmon fillets on the prepared baking sheet. Season with salt and pepper.
3. In a small bowl, combine minced garlic, chopped parsley, chopped dill, and olive oil. Mix well.
4. Spread the herb mixture evenly over the salmon fillets.
5. Arrange lemon slices on top of the salmon.

6. Bake in the preheated oven for 12-15 minutes, or until salmon is cooked through and flakes easily with a fork.

7. Serve baked lemon herb salmon hot, garnished with lemon wedges if desired.

8. Enjoy this flavorful and nutritious dinner!

Nutrition Facts (per serving):

- Calories: 300
- Total Fat: 15g
- Saturated Fat: 2g
- Cholesterol: 80mg
- Sodium: 120mg
- Total Carbohydrates: 2g
- Dietary Fiber: 1g
- Sugars: 0g
- Protein: 38g

Turkey and Vegetable Stir-Fry

Prep Time: 15 mins

Cook Time: 15 mins

Total Time: 30 mins

Servings: 2

Ingredients:

- 1/2 lb ground turkey
- 2 cups mixed vegetables (bell peppers, snap peas, carrots)
- 2 cloves garlic, minced
- 1 tablespoon grated ginger

- 2 tablespoons low-sodium soy sauce

- 1 tablespoon sesame oil

- 1 tablespoon honey or maple syrup

- Salt and pepper to taste

- Optional garnish: chopped green onions, sesame seeds

Directions:

1. Heat sesame oil in a large skillet or wok over medium-high heat.

2. Add minced garlic and grated ginger to the skillet. Stir-fry for 1 minute until fragrant.

3. Add ground turkey to the skillet. Cook, breaking it apart with a spatula, until browned and cooked through, about 5-6 minutes.

4. Add mixed vegetables to the skillet. Stir-fry for 3-4 minutes until vegetables are tender-crisp.

5. In a small bowl, mix soy sauce and honey or maple syrup to make the sauce.

6. Pour the sauce over the turkey and vegetables in the skillet. Stir until everything is evenly coated and heated through.

7. Season with salt and pepper to taste.

8. Serve turkey and vegetable stir-fry hot, garnished with chopped green onions and sesame seeds if desired.

9. Enjoy this protein-rich and flavorful dinner!

Nutrition Facts (per serving):

- Calories: 280

- Total Fat: 10g

- Saturated Fat: 2g

- Cholesterol: 60mg

- Sodium: 480mg

- Total Carbohydrates: 20g

- Dietary Fiber: 4g

- Sugars: 10g

- Protein: 26g

Vegetarian Lentil Soup

Prep Time: 10 mins

Cook Time: 40 mins

Total Time: 50 mins

Servings: 4

Ingredients:

- 1 cup dry green lentils, rinsed and drained

- 4 cups low-sodium vegetable broth

- 1 onion, diced

- 2 carrots, diced

- 2 stalks celery, diced

- 2 cloves garlic, minced

- 1 teaspoon ground cumin

- 1/2 teaspoon smoked paprika

- Salt and pepper to taste

- 2 tablespoons chopped fresh parsley

- Optional: lemon wedges for serving

Directions:

1. In a large pot, combine green lentils, vegetable broth, diced onion, diced carrots, diced celery, minced garlic, ground cumin, and smoked paprika.

2. Bring the mixture to a boil over medium-high heat. Reduce heat to low, cover, and simmer for 30-35 minutes, or until lentils and vegetables are tender.

3. Season with salt and pepper to taste.

4. Stir in chopped fresh parsley.

5. Ladle vegetarian lentil soup into bowls. Serve hot, garnished with lemon wedges if desired.

6. Enjoy this hearty and comforting soup!

Nutrition Facts (per serving):

- Calories: 220
- Total Fat: 1g
- Saturated Fat: 0g
- Cholesterol: 0mg
- Sodium: 490mg
- Total Carbohydrates: 38g
- Dietary Fiber: 16g
- Sugars: 4g
- Protein: 14g

Baked Chicken with Roasted Vegetables

Prep Time: 15 mins

Cook Time: 30 mins

Total Time: 45 mins

Servings: 2

Ingredients:

- 2 boneless, skinless chicken breasts
- 2 cups mixed vegetables (zucchini, bell peppers, onions)
- 2 tablespoons olive oil
- 2 cloves garlic, minced
- 1 teaspoon dried thyme
- 1 teaspoon dried rosemary
- Salt and pepper to taste
- Optional: lemon wedges for serving

Directions:

1. Preheat oven to 400°F (200°C). Line a baking sheet with parchment paper.
2. Place chicken breasts on one side of the prepared baking sheet.
3. In a mixing bowl, toss mixed vegetables with olive oil, minced garlic, dried thyme, dried rosemary, salt, and pepper until evenly coated.
4. Spread the seasoned vegetables on the other side of the baking sheet.
5. Bake in the preheated oven for 25-30 minutes, or until chicken is cooked through and vegetables are tender and lightly browned.
6. Serve baked chicken with roasted vegetables hot, garnished with lemon wedges if desired.
7. Enjoy this wholesome and satisfying meal!

Nutrition Facts (per serving):

- Calories: 320
- Total Fat: 14g
- Saturated Fat: 2g
- Cholesterol: 80mg
- Sodium: 180mg
- Total Carbohydrates: 14g
- Dietary Fiber: 5g
- Sugars: 5g
- Protein: 34g

Lemon Garlic Shrimp with Quinoa

Prep Time: 10 mins

Cook Time: 20 mins

Total Time: 30 mins

Servings: 2

Ingredients:

- 1/2 cup quinoa
- 1 cup water or low-sodium vegetable broth
- 1 tablespoon olive oil
- 1/2 lb shrimp, peeled and deveined
- 2 cloves garlic, minced
- 1 tablespoon chopped fresh parsley
- 1 tablespoon lemon juice
- Salt and pepper to taste
- Optional: lemon wedges for serving

Directions:

1. Rinse quinoa under cold water and drain.

2. In a saucepan, bring water or vegetable broth to a boil. Add quinoa, reduce heat to low, cover, and simmer for 15 minutes, or until quinoa is tender and liquid is absorbed. Remove from heat and let it cool slightly.

3. Heat olive oil in a skillet over medium heat. Add minced garlic and cook for 1 minute until fragrant.

4. Add shrimp to the skillet and cook until pink and opaque, about 2-3 minutes per side.

5. Stir in cooked quinoa, chopped parsley, and lemon juice. Season with salt and pepper to taste.

6. Cook for another 2 minutes, stirring occasionally.

7. Serve lemon garlic shrimp with quinoa hot, garnished with lemon wedges if desired.

8. Enjoy this light and flavorful dinner!

Nutrition Facts (per serving):

- Calories: 320
- Total Fat: 9g
- Saturated Fat: 1g
- Cholesterol: 120mg
- Sodium: 210mg
- Total Carbohydrates: 34g
- Dietary Fiber: 4g
- Sugars: 1g
- Protein: 28g

Turkey and Vegetable Skillet

Prep Time: 10 mins

Cook Time: 20 mins

Total Time: 30 mins

Servings: 2

Ingredients:

- 1/2 lb ground turkey
- 1 tablespoon olive oil
- 1 onion, diced
- 2 cloves garlic, minced
- 1 bell pepper, diced
- 1 zucchini, diced
- 1 cup cherry tomatoes, halved
- 1 teaspoon Italian seasoning
- Salt and pepper to taste
- Optional: grated Parmesan cheese for serving

Directions:

1. Heat olive oil in a skillet over medium-high heat. Add diced onion and minced garlic. Cook until softened and fragrant, about 2-3 minutes.

2. Add ground turkey to the skillet. Cook, breaking it apart with a spatula, until browned and cooked through, about 5-6 minutes.

3. Add diced bell pepper and zucchini to the skillet. Cook for 3-4 minutes until vegetables are tender-crisp.

4. Stir in cherry tomatoes, Italian seasoning, salt, and pepper. Cook for another 2-3 minutes until tomatoes are softened.

5. Serve turkey and vegetable skillet hot, garnished with grated Parmesan cheese if desired.

6. Enjoy this wholesome and nutritious dinner!

Nutrition Facts (per serving):

- Calories: 280
- Total Fat: 14g
- Saturated Fat: 3g
- Cholesterol: 60mg
- Sodium: 320mg
- Total Carbohydrates: 16g
- Dietary Fiber: 5g
- Sugars: 8g
- Protein: 24g

Baked Cod with Roasted Vegetables

Prep Time: 15 mins

Cook Time: 20 mins

Total Time: 35 mins

Servings: 2

Ingredients:

- 2 cod fillets
- 2 cups mixed vegetables (broccoli, cauliflower, carrots)
- 2 tablespoons olive oil
- 2 cloves garlic, minced
- 1 teaspoon dried thyme
- 1 teaspoon dried rosemary

- Salt and pepper to taste
- Optional: lemon wedges for serving

Directions:

1. Preheat oven to 400°F (200°C). Line a baking sheet with parchment paper.
2. Place cod fillets on one side of the prepared baking sheet.
3. In a mixing bowl, toss mixed vegetables with olive oil, minced garlic, dried thyme, dried rosemary, salt, and pepper until evenly coated.
4. Spread the seasoned vegetables on the other side of the baking sheet.
5. Bake in the preheated oven for 15-20 minutes, or until cod is cooked through and vegetables are tender and lightly browned.
6. Serve baked cod with roasted vegetables hot, garnished with lemon wedges if desired.
7. Enjoy this simple and satisfying dinner!

Nutrition Facts (per serving):

- Calories: 300
- Total Fat: 12g
- Saturated Fat: 2g
- Cholesterol: 60mg
- Sodium: 280mg
- Total Carbohydrates: 20g
- Dietary Fiber: 6g
- Sugars: 6g
- Protein: 30g

Vegetarian Stuffed Bell Peppers

Prep Time: 20 mins

Cook Time: 40 mins

Total Time: 1 hour

Servings: 2

Ingredients:

- 2 large bell peppers (any color)
- 1/2 cup quinoa
- 1 cup water or low-sodium vegetable broth
- 1 tablespoon olive oil
- 1 onion, diced
- 2 cloves garlic, minced
- 1 zucchini, diced
- 1 cup cherry tomatoes, halved
- 1/4 cup chopped fresh parsley
- 1/4 cup grated Parmesan cheese
- Salt and pepper to taste

Directions:

1. Preheat oven to 375°F (190°C). Grease a baking dish.
2. Cut the tops off the bell peppers and remove the seeds and membranes.
3. In a saucepan, bring water or vegetable broth to a boil. Add quinoa, reduce heat to low, cover, and simmer for 15 minutes, or until quinoa is tender and liquid is absorbed. Remove from heat and let it cool slightly.

4. Heat olive oil in a skillet over medium heat. Add diced onion and minced garlic. Cook until softened and fragrant, about 2-3 minutes.

5. Add diced zucchini and cherry tomatoes to the skillet. Cook for 3-4 minutes until vegetables are tender-crisp.

6. Stir in cooked quinoa, chopped parsley, and grated Parmesan cheese. Season with salt and pepper to taste.

7. Stuff the bell peppers with the quinoa and vegetable mixture.

8. Place stuffed bell peppers in the prepared baking dish. Cover with aluminum foil and bake in the preheated oven for 30-35 minutes, or until peppers are tender.

9. Serve vegetarian stuffed bell peppers hot.

10. Enjoy this colorful and nutritious dinner!

Nutrition Facts (per serving):

- Calories: 290
- Total Fat: 10g
- Saturated Fat: 3g
- Cholesterol: 10mg
- Sodium: 300mg
- Total Carbohydrates: 40g
- Dietary Fiber: 8g
- Sugars: 10g
- Protein: 12g

Grilled Lemon Herb Chicken Breast

Prep Time: 10 mins

Cook Time: 15 mins

Total Time: 25 mins

Servings: 2

Ingredients:

- 2 boneless, skinless chicken breasts
- 2 tablespoons olive oil
- 2 cloves garlic, minced
- Zest and juice of 1 lemon
- 1 tablespoon chopped fresh parsley
- 1 tablespoon chopped fresh thyme
- Salt and pepper to taste
- Optional: lemon wedges for serving

Directions:

1. Preheat grill to medium-high heat.
2. In a small bowl, whisk together olive oil, minced garlic, lemon zest, lemon juice, chopped parsley, chopped thyme, salt, and pepper to make the marinade.
3. Place chicken breasts in a shallow dish and pour the marinade over them. Make sure the chicken is evenly coated. Let it marinate for at least 30 minutes.
4. Remove chicken from the marinade and discard excess marinade.
5. Grill chicken breasts for 6-7 minutes per side, or until cooked through and no longer pink in the center.

6. Remove from the grill and let the chicken rest for a few minutes before serving.

7. Serve grilled lemon herb chicken breast hot, garnished with lemon wedges if desired.

8. Enjoy this flavorful and protein-packed dinner!

Nutrition Facts (per serving):

- Calories: 250

- Total Fat: 12g

- Saturated Fat: 2g

- Cholesterol: 80mg

- Sodium: 110mg

- Total Carbohydrates: 2g

- Dietary Fiber: 1g

- Sugars: 0g

- Protein: 32g

Salmon and Asparagus Foil Packets

Prep Time: 10 mins

Cook Time: 20 mins

Total Time: 30 mins

Servings: 2

Ingredients:

- 2 salmon fillets

- 1 bunch asparagus, trimmed

- 2 tablespoons olive oil

- 2 cloves garlic, minced

- Zest and juice of 1 lemon
- Salt and pepper to taste

Directions:

1. Preheat oven to 400°F (200°C).
2. Cut two large pieces of aluminum foil.
3. Place one salmon fillet in the center of each piece of foil.
4. Arrange asparagus spears around the salmon fillets.
5. In a small bowl, whisk together olive oil, minced garlic, lemon zest, lemon juice, salt, and pepper to make the marinade.
6. Drizzle the marinade over the salmon and asparagus.
7. Fold the sides of the foil over the salmon and asparagus, sealing the edges to create a packet.
8. Place the foil packets on a baking sheet and bake in the preheated oven for 15-20 minutes, or until salmon is cooked through and asparagus is tender.
9. Carefully open the foil packets and transfer the salmon and asparagus to serving plates.
10. Serve salmon and asparagus foil packets hot.
11. Enjoy this simple and delicious dinner!

Nutrition Facts (per serving):

- Calories: 300
- Total Fat: 18g
- Saturated Fat: 3g
- Cholesterol: 80mg
- Sodium: 120mg
- Total Carbohydrates: 5g

- Dietary Fiber: 3g

- Sugars: 2g

- Protein: 30g

Mediterranean Quinoa Salad

Prep Time: 15 mins

Cook Time: 15 mins

Total Time: 30 mins

Servings: 2

Ingredients:

- 1/2 cup quinoa

- 1 cup water or low-sodium vegetable broth

- 1 cup cherry tomatoes, halved

- 1/2 cucumber, diced

- 1/4 cup chopped red onion

- 1/4 cup chopped fresh parsley

- 2 tablespoons chopped fresh mint

- 2 tablespoons olive oil

- 1 tablespoon lemon juice

- Salt and pepper to taste

- Optional: crumbled feta cheese for serving

Directions:

1. Rinse quinoa under cold water and drain.

2. In a saucepan, bring water or vegetable broth to a boil. Add quinoa, reduce heat to low, cover, and simmer for 15 minutes, or until quinoa is tender and liquid is absorbed. Remove from heat and let it cool slightly.

3. In a large bowl, combine cooked quinoa, cherry tomatoes, diced cucumber, chopped red onion, chopped parsley, and chopped mint.

4. In a small bowl, whisk together olive oil, lemon juice, salt, and pepper to make the dressing.

5. Drizzle the dressing over the quinoa salad and toss to coat evenly.

6. Serve Mediterranean quinoa salad chilled or at room temperature, garnished with crumbled feta cheese if desired.

7. Enjoy this refreshing and nutritious salad!

Nutrition Facts (per serving):

- Calories: 280
- Total Fat: 14g
- Saturated Fat: 2g
- Cholesterol: 0mg
- Sodium: 200mg
- Total Carbohydrates: 32g
- Dietary Fiber: 5g
- Sugars: 3g
- Protein: 6g

Vegetable and Chickpea Curry

Prep Time: 15 mins

Cook Time: 25 mins

Total Time: 40 mins

Servings: 2

Ingredients:

- 1 tablespoon olive oil
- 1 onion, diced
- 2 cloves garlic, minced
- 1 tablespoon grated ginger
- 1 tablespoon curry powder
- 1 teaspoon ground turmeric
- 1 can (14 oz.) chickpeas, drained and rinsed
- 1 can (14 oz) diced tomatoes
- 2 cups mixed vegetables (such as bell peppers, carrots, and cauliflower), chopped
- 1 cup coconut milk
- Salt and pepper to taste
- Fresh cilantro for garnish

Directions:

1. Heat olive oil in a large skillet over medium heat. Add diced onion and cook until softened, about 5 minutes.
2. Add minced garlic, grated ginger, curry powder, and ground turmeric to the skillet. Cook for 1-2 minutes until fragrant.
3. Stir in drained chickpeas, diced tomatoes, and mixed vegetables. Cook for 5 minutes, stirring occasionally.
4. Pour in coconut milk and bring the mixture to a simmer. Reduce heat to low and let it simmer for 10-15 minutes, or until vegetables are tender and the curry has thickened slightly.
5. Season with salt and pepper to taste.

6. Serve vegetable and chickpea curry hot, garnished with fresh cilantro.

7. Enjoy this comforting and flavorful dinner!

Nutrition Facts (per serving):

- Calories: 350
- Total Fat: 16g
- Saturated Fat: 9g
- Cholesterol: 0mg
- Sodium: 480mg
- Total Carbohydrates: 46g
- Dietary Fiber: 11g
- Sugars: 12g
- Protein: 9g

Grilled Lemon Herb Salmon

Prep Time: 10 mins

Cook Time: 10 mins

Total Time: 20 mins

Servings: 2

Ingredients:

- 2 salmon fillets
- 2 tablespoons olive oil
- 1 lemon, thinly sliced
- 2 cloves garlic, minced
- 1 tablespoon chopped fresh parsley
- 1 tablespoon chopped fresh dill

- Salt and pepper to taste

Directions:

1. Preheat grill to medium-high heat.
2. Brush salmon fillets with olive oil and season with salt and pepper.
3. Place lemon slices on top of each salmon fillet.
4. In a small bowl, mix together minced garlic, chopped parsley, and chopped dill.
5. Sprinkle the herb mixture over the salmon fillets.
6. Grill salmon for 4-5 minutes on each side, or until fish flakes easily with a fork.
7. Remove from grill and serve immediately.
8. Enjoy this delicious and nutritious grilled salmon!

Nutrition Facts (per serving):

- Calories: 300
- Total Fat: 20g
- Saturated Fat: 3g
- Cholesterol: 80mg
- Sodium: 90mg
- Total Carbohydrates: 2g
- Dietary Fiber: 1g
- Sugars: 0g
- Protein: 28g

Turkey and Vegetable Stir-Fry

Prep Time: 15 mins

Cook Time: 15 mins

Total Time: 30 mins

Servings: 2

Ingredients:

- 1 tablespoon olive oil
- 1 pound turkey breast, sliced
- 1 bell pepper, sliced
- 1 cup broccoli florets
- 1 cup snap peas
- 2 cloves garlic, minced
- 2 tablespoons low-sodium soy sauce
- 1 tablespoon rice vinegar
- 1 teaspoon sesame oil
- 1 teaspoon honey
- Sesame seeds for garnish (optional)

Directions:

1. Heat olive oil in a large skillet or wok over medium-high heat.

2. Add sliced turkey breast to the skillet and cook until browned and cooked through, about 5-7 minutes. Remove from skillet and set aside.

3. In the same skillet, add bell pepper, broccoli florets, snap peas, and minced garlic. Stir-fry for 3-4 minutes, or until vegetables are tender-crisp.

4. Return cooked turkey to the skillet with the vegetables.

5. In a small bowl, whisk together low-sodium soy sauce, rice vinegar, sesame oil, and honey. Pour the sauce over the turkey and vegetables in the skillet.

6. Stir-fry for another 2-3 minutes, until everything is heated through and evenly coated with the sauce.

7. Remove from heat and garnish with sesame seeds if desired.

8. Serve turkey and vegetable stir-fry hot over brown rice or quinoa.

9. Enjoy this flavorful and protein-rich stir-fry!

Nutrition Facts (per serving):

- Calories: 280
- Total Fat: 8g
- Saturated Fat: 1
- Cholesterol: 70mg
- Sodium: 500mg
- Total Carbohydrates: 15g
- Dietary Fiber: 4g
- Sugars: 6g
- Protein: 38g

Vegetable and Lentil Soup

Prep Time: 15 mins

Cook Time: 30 mins

Total Time: 45 mins

Servings: 4

Ingredients:

- 1 tablespoon olive oil
- 1 onion, diced
- 2 carrots, diced
- 2 stalks celery, diced
- 2 cloves garlic, minced
- 1 cup dried green lentils, rinsed and drained
- 4 cups low-sodium vegetable broth
- 1 can (14 oz) diced tomatoes
- 1 teaspoon dried thyme
- 1 teaspoon dried oregano
- Salt and pepper to taste
- Fresh parsley for garnish

Directions:

1. Heat olive oil in a large pot over medium heat.
2. Add diced onion, carrots, and celery to the pot. Cook until vegetables are softened, about 5-7 minutes.
3. Add minced garlic to the pot and cook for another 1-2 minutes, until fragrant.
4. Stir in dried green lentils, low-sodium vegetable broth, diced tomatoes, dried thyme, and dried oregano. Bring to a boil.
5. Reduce heat to low, cover, and simmer for 20-25 minutes, or until lentils are tender.
6. Season with salt and pepper to taste.
7. Serve vegetable and lentil soup hot, garnished with fresh parsley.
8. Enjoy this hearty and comforting soup!

Nutrition Facts (per serving):

- Calories: 250
- Total Fat: 4g
- Saturated Fat: 1g
- Cholesterol: 0mg
- Sodium: 350mg
- Total Carbohydrates: 40g
- Dietary Fiber: 15g
- Sugars: 8g
- Protein: 15g

Baked Lemon Herb Chicken with Roasted Vegetables

Prep Time: 15 mins

Cook Time: 30 mins

Total Time: 45 mins

Servings: 2

Ingredients:

- 2 boneless, skinless chicken breasts
- 2 tablespoons olive oil
- Zest and juice of 1 lemon
- 1 teaspoon dried thyme
- 1 teaspoon dried rosemary
- 1 teaspoon dried oregano
- Salt and pepper to taste
- 1 sweet potato, peeled and diced
- 1 zucchini, sliced

- 1 red bell pepper, sliced
- 1 tablespoon balsamic vinegar

Directions:

1. Preheat oven to 400°F (200°C).
2. Place chicken breasts in a baking dish.
3. In a small bowl, whisk together olive oil, lemon zest, lemon juice, dried thyme, dried rosemary, dried oregano, salt, and pepper. Pour the marinade over the chicken breasts, turning to coat evenly.
4. In a separate baking dish, toss diced sweet potato, sliced zucchini, and sliced red bell pepper with olive oil, salt, and pepper.
5. Place both baking dishes in the preheated oven. Bake chicken for 25-30 minutes, or until cooked through and no longer pink in the center. Bake vegetables for 20-25 minutes, or until tender and lightly browned.
6. Remove from oven and let chicken rest for a few minutes before slicing.
7. Drizzle roasted vegetables with balsamic vinegar before serving.
8. Serve baked lemon herb chicken with roasted vegetables hot.
9. Enjoy this satisfying and wholesome dinner!

Nutrition Facts (per serving):

- Calories: 320
- Total Fat: 12g
- Saturated Fat: 2g

- Cholesterol: 80mg

- Sodium: 400mg

- Total Carbohydrates: 20g

- Dietary Fiber: 5g

- Sugars: 6g

- Protein: 35g

SNACKS RECIPES

Hummus and Veggie Snack Plate

Prep Time: 10 mins

Total Time: 10 mins

Servings: 2

Ingredients:

- 1 cup baby carrots
- 1 cup cucumber slices
- 1 cup cherry tomatoes
- 1/2 cup hummus
- Fresh parsley for garnish
- Whole grain crackers or rice cakes (optional)

Directions:

1. Wash and prepare the vegetables by cutting baby carrots into sticks, slicing cucumbers, and halving cherry tomatoes.
2. Arrange the vegetables on a plate along with a dollop of hummus.
3. Garnish with fresh parsley.
4. Serve with whole grain crackers or rice cakes if desired.
5. Enjoy this nutritious and satisfying snack!

Nutrition Facts (per serving):

- Calories: 150
- Total Fat: 6g
- Saturated Fat: 1g
- Cholesterol: 0mg

- Sodium: 300mg

- Total Carbohydrates: 20g

- Dietary Fiber: 7g

- Sugars: 7g

- Protein: 6g

Greek Yogurt Parfait with Berries

Prep Time: 5 mins

Total Time: 5 mins

Servings: 2

Ingredients:

- 1 cup Greek yogurt

- 1/2 cup mixed berries (such as strawberries, blueberries, raspberries)

- 2 tablespoons chopped nuts (such as almonds, walnuts)

- 1 tablespoon honey or maple syrup (optional)

Directions:

1. In two serving glasses or bowls, layer Greek yogurt, mixed berries, and chopped nuts.

2. Drizzle with honey or maple syrup if desired.

3. Serve immediately or refrigerate until ready to eat.

4. Enjoy this delicious and protein-packed snack!

Nutrition Facts (per serving):

- Calories: 200

- Total Fat: 8g

- Saturated Fat: 1g

- Cholesterol: 5mg

- Sodium: 50mg

- Total Carbohydrates: 20g

- Dietary Fiber: 3g

- Sugars: 14g

- Protein: 12g

Avocado Toast with Tomato and Basil

Prep Time: 5 mins

Total Time: 5 mins

Servings: 2

Ingredients:

- 2 slices whole grain bread, toasted

- 1 ripe avocado

- 1 tomato, sliced

- Fresh basil leaves

- Salt and pepper to taste

- Red pepper flakes (optional)

Directions:

1. Mash the ripe avocado in a bowl and season with salt and pepper.

2. Spread mashed avocado evenly onto each slice of toasted whole grain bread.

3. Top with sliced tomatoes and fresh basil leaves.

4. Sprinkle with red pepper flakes if desired.

5. Serve immediately.

6. Enjoy this simple yet delicious snack!

Nutrition Facts (per serving):

- Calories: 180
- Total Fat: 10g
- Saturated Fat: 1.5g
- Cholesterol: 0mg
- Sodium: 200mg
- Total Carbohydrates: 20g
- Dietary Fiber: 7g
- Sugars: 3g
- Protein: 5g

Cottage Cheese and Pineapple

Prep Time: 5 mins

Total Time: 5 mins

Servings: 2

Ingredients:

- 1 cup low-fat cottage cheese
- 1 cup fresh pineapple chunks

Directions:

1. Divide the low-fat cottage cheese and fresh pineapple chunks between two serving bowls.
2. Serve immediately.
3. Enjoy this protein-rich and refreshing snack!

Nutrition Facts (per serving):

- Calories: 150

- Total Fat: 2g

- Saturated Fat: 1g

- Cholesterol: 10mg

- Sodium: 300mg

- Total Carbohydrates: 20g

- Dietary Fiber: 2g

- Sugars: 15g

- Protein: 15g

Quinoa Salad with Chickpeas and Vegetables

Prep Time: 10 mins

Total Time: 20 mins

Servings: 2

Ingredients:

- 1/2 cup quinoa

- 1 cup water or vegetable broth

- 1 can (15 oz.) chickpeas, drained and rinsed

- 1 cucumber, diced

- 1 bell pepper, diced

- 1/4 cup chopped fresh parsley

- 2 tablespoons lemon juice

- 2 tablespoons olive oil

- Salt and pepper to taste

Directions:

1. Rinse quinoa under cold water. In a medium saucepan, combine quinoa and water or vegetable broth. Bring to a boil, then

reduce heat to low, cover, and simmer for 15 minutes, or until quinoa is tender and liquid is absorbed. Remove from heat and let it cool.

2. In a large bowl, combine cooked quinoa, chickpeas, cucumber, bell pepper, and chopped parsley.

3. In a small bowl, whisk together lemon juice, olive oil, salt, and pepper. Pour dressing over the salad and toss to combine.

4. Serve immediately or refrigerate until ready to eat.

5. Enjoy this nutritious and flavorful snack!

Nutrition Facts (per serving):

- Calories: 320
- Total Fat: 10g
- Saturated Fat: 1g
- Cholesterol: 0mg
- Sodium: 380mg
- Total Carbohydrates: 48g
- Dietary Fiber: 10g
- Sugars: 6g
- Protein: 12g

Greek Yogurt with Berries and Almonds

Prep Time: 5 mins

Total Time: 5 mins

Servings: 2

Ingredients:

- 1 cup Greek yogurt

- 1/2 cup mixed berries (such as strawberries, blueberries, raspberries)
- 1/4 cup sliced almonds
- 1 tablespoon honey or maple syrup (optional)

Directions:

1. In two serving bowls, divide Greek yogurt.
2. Top with mixed berries and sliced almonds.
3. Drizzle with honey or maple syrup if desired.
4. Serve immediately.
5. Enjoy this protein-rich and satisfying snack!

Nutrition Facts (per serving):

- Calories: 250
- Total Fat: 10g
- Saturated Fat: 1g
- Cholesterol: 10mg
- Sodium: 50mg
- Total Carbohydrates: 20g
- Dietary Fiber: 3g
- Sugars: 14g
- Protein: 12g

Crispy Kale Chips

Prep Time: 10 mins

Total Time: 25 mins

Servings: 2

Ingredients:

- 1 bunch kale, stems removed and leaves torn into bite-sized pieces
- 1 tablespoon olive oil
- Salt and pepper to taste

Directions:

1. Preheat oven to 300°F (150°C).
2. In a large bowl, toss kale leaves with olive oil, salt, and pepper until evenly coated.
3. Spread kale leaves in a single layer on a baking sheet.
4. Bake for 20-25 minutes, or until kale is crispy but not burnt, stirring halfway through.
5. Remove from oven and let cool before serving.
6. Enjoy this crunchy and nutritious snack!

Nutrition Facts (per serving):

- Calories: 100
- Total Fat: 7g
- Saturated Fat: 1g
- Cholesterol: 0mg
- Sodium: 30mg
- Total Carbohydrates: 8g
- Dietary Fiber: 2g
- Sugars: 1g
- Protein: 4g

Smoked Salmon Cucumber Bites

Prep Time: 10 mins

Total Time: 10 mins

Servings: 2

Ingredients:

- 1 English cucumber, cut into slices
- 4 oz smoked salmon, sliced
- 2 tablespoons cream cheese
- Fresh dill for garnish

Directions:

1. Place cucumber slices on a serving plate.
2. Top each cucumber slice with a small piece of smoked salmon.
3. Dollop a small amount of cream cheese on top of the salmon.
4. Garnish with fresh dill.
5. Serve immediately.
6. Enjoy this elegant and protein-packed snack!

Nutrition Facts (per serving):

- Calories: 150
- Total Fat: 8g
- Saturated Fat: 3g
- Cholesterol: 25mg
- Sodium: 300mg
- Total Carbohydrates: 5g
- Dietary Fiber: 1g
- Sugars: 2g
- Protein: 15g

Apple Slices with Almond Butter

Prep Time: 5 mins

Total Time: 5 mins

Servings: 2

Ingredients:

- 1 apple, sliced
- 2 tablespoons almond butter
- Cinnamon for sprinkling (optional)

Directions:

1. Arrange apple slices on a plate.
2. Serve almond butter on the side for dipping.
3. Sprinkle with cinnamon if desired.
4. Enjoy this simple and satisfying snack!

Nutrition Facts (per serving):

- Calories: 200
- Total Fat: 12g
- Saturated Fat: 1g
- Cholesterol: 0mg
- Sodium: 0mg
- Total Carbohydrates: 22g
- Dietary Fiber: 5g
- Sugars: 15g
- Protein: 5g

Baked Sweet Potato Fries

Ingredients:

- 2 medium sweet potatoes
- 1 tablespoon olive oil
- 1/2 teaspoon paprika
- 1/2 teaspoon garlic powder
- Salt and pepper to taste

Directions:

1. Preheat oven to 425°F (220°C). Line a baking sheet with parchment paper.
2. Peel the sweet potatoes and cut them into fry's shape.
3. In a large bowl, toss the sweet potato fries with olive oil, paprika, garlic powder, salt, and pepper until evenly coated.
4. Spread the fries in a single layer on the prepared baking sheet.
5. Bake for 25-30 minutes, flipping halfway through, until fries are golden and crispy.
6. Remove from the oven and let cool for a few minutes before serving.
7. Enjoy these crunchy and flavorful sweet potato fries!

Nutrition Facts (per serving):

- Calories: 180
- Total Fat: 5g
- Saturated Fat: 1g
- Cholesterol: 0mg

- Sodium: 70mg

- Total Carbohydrates: 32g

- Dietary Fiber: 5g

- Sugars: 6g

- Protein: 3g

Hummus with Veggie Sticks

Prep Time: 10 mins

Total Time: 10 mins

Servings: 2

Ingredients:

- 1/2 cup hummus

- 1 carrot, cut into sticks

- 1 cucumber, cut into sticks

- 1 bell pepper, sliced

- 1 stalk celery, cut into sticks

Directions:

1. Place hummus in a serving bowl.

2. Arrange carrot sticks, cucumber sticks, bell pepper slices, and celery sticks around the hummus.

3. Serve immediately.

4. Enjoy this crunchy and protein-rich snack!

Nutrition Facts (per serving):

- Calories: 150

- Total Fat: 7g

- Saturated Fat: 1g

- Cholesterol: 0mg

- Sodium: 300mg

- Total Carbohydrates: 18g

- Dietary Fiber: 6g

- Sugars: 3g

- Protein: 6g

Avocado Toast with Tomato

Prep Time: 5 mins

Total Time: 10 mins

Servings: 2

Ingredients:

- 2 slices whole grain bread, toasted

- 1 ripe avocado

- 1 small tomato, sliced

- Salt and pepper to taste

- Red pepper flakes for garnish (optional)

- Lemon juice (optional)

Directions:

1. Mash the avocado in a small bowl with a fork. Season with salt, pepper, and a squeeze of lemon juice if desired.

2. Spread mashed avocado evenly on toasted bread slices.

3. Top with sliced tomatoes.

4. Sprinkle with red pepper flakes if desired.

5. Serve immediately.

6. Enjoy this creamy and nutritious snack!

Nutrition Facts (per serving):

- Calories: 200
- Total Fat: 10g
- Saturated Fat: 1g
- Cholesterol: 0mg
- Sodium: 150mg
- Total Carbohydrates: 24g
- Dietary Fiber: 7g
- Sugars: 2g
- Protein: 6g

Cottage Cheese with Pineapple

Prep Time: 5 mins

Total Time: 5 mins

Servings: 2

Ingredients:

- 1 cup cottage cheese
- 1 cup fresh pineapple chunks

Directions:

1. Divide cottage cheese into serving bowls.
2. Top with fresh pineapple chunks.
3. Serve immediately.
4. Enjoy this protein-packed and refreshing snack!

Nutrition Facts (per serving):

- Calories: 150
- Total Fat: 2g

- Saturated Fat: 1g

- Cholesterol: 10mg

- Sodium: 400mg

- Total Carbohydrates: 16g

- Dietary Fiber: 1g

- Sugars: 14g

- Protein: 15g

Stuffed Bell Peppers

Prep Time: 15 mins

Total Time: 40 mins

Servings: 2

Ingredients:

- 2 large bell peppers (any color)

- 1/2 cup cooked quinoa

- 1/2 cup black beans, drained and rinsed

- 1/2 cup corn kernels (fresh or frozen)

- 1/4 cup diced tomatoes

- 1/4 cup chopped fresh cilantro

- 1/2 teaspoon cumin

- 1/2 teaspoon chili powder

- Salt and pepper to taste

- 1/4 cup shredded cheese (optional)

Directions:

1. Preheat oven to 375°F (190°C). Grease a baking dish.

2. Cut the tops off the bell peppers and remove seeds and membranes.

3. In a large bowl, mix together cooked quinoa, black beans, corn, diced tomatoes, cilantro, cumin, chili powder, salt, and pepper.

4. Spoon the quinoa mixture into the bell peppers, packing tightly.

5. Place stuffed bell peppers in the prepared baking dish. If desired, sprinkle shredded cheese on top.

6. Bake for 25-30 minutes, or until bell peppers are tender.

7. Remove from oven and let cool for a few minutes before serving.

8. Enjoy these flavorful and nutritious stuffed bell peppers!

Nutrition Facts (per serving):

- Calories: 250Total Fat: 3g
- Saturated Fat: 1g
- Cholesterol: 5mg
- Sodium: 450mg
- Total Carbohydrates: 45g
- Dietary Fiber: 9g
- Sugars: 10g
- Protein: 11g

Quinoa Salad with Avocado and Chickpeas

Prep Time: 10 mins

Total Time: 25 mins

Servings: 2

Ingredients:

- 1/2 cup quinoa

- 1 cup water or vegetable broth

- 1 avocado, diced

- 1/2 cup canned chickpeas, drained and rinsed

- 1/4 cup diced cucumber

- 1/4 cup diced bell pepper

- 2 tablespoons chopped fresh cilantro

- 1 tablespoon olive oil

- 1 tablespoon lemon juice

- Salt and pepper to taste

Directions:

1. Rinse quinoa under cold water. In a small saucepan, bring water or vegetable broth to a boil. Add quinoa, reduce heat to low, cover, and simmer for 15 minutes, or until quinoa is cooked and liquid is absorbed. Remove from heat and let cool.

2. In a large bowl, combine cooked quinoa, diced avocado, chickpeas, cucumber, bell pepper, and cilantro.

3. In a small bowl, whisk together olive oil, lemon juice, salt, and pepper. Pour dressing over the salad and toss to coat evenly.

4. Serve immediately or chill in the refrigerator for a refreshing snack or light meal.

Nutrition Facts (per serving):

- Calories: 320

- Total Fat: 16g

- Saturated Fat: 2g

- Cholesterol: 0mg

- Sodium: 10mg

- Total Carbohydrates: 40g

- Dietary Fiber: 11g

- Sugars: 2g

- Protein: 9g

Greek Yogurt Parfait

Prep Time: 5 mins

Total Time: 5 mins

Servings: 1

Ingredients:

- 1/2 cup Greek yogurt

- 1/4 cup granola

- 1/4 cup mixed berries (such as strawberries, blueberries, raspberries)

- 1 tablespoon honey (optional)

Directions:

1. In a serving glass or bowl, layer Greek yogurt, granola, and mixed berries.

2. Drizzle honey on top if desired.

3. Serve immediately and enjoy this delicious and protein-rich snack!

Nutrition Facts (per serving):

- Calories: 250

- Total Fat: 5g

- Saturated Fat: 0.5g

- Cholesterol: 5mg

- Sodium: 50mg

- Total Carbohydrates: 40g

- Dietary Fiber: 5g

- Sugars: 20g

- Protein: 15g

Cucumber Slices with Tzatziki

Prep Time: 10 mins

Total Time: 10 mins

Servings: 2

Ingredients:

- 1 medium cucumber

- 1/2 cup Greek yogurt

- 1 clove garlic, minced

- 1 tablespoon chopped fresh dill

- 1 tablespoon lemon juice

- Salt and pepper to taste

Directions:

1. Slice the cucumber into thin rounds.

2. In a small bowl, mix together Greek yogurt, minced garlic, chopped fresh dill, lemon juice, salt, and pepper to make the tzatziki sauce.

3. Serve cucumber slices with tzatziki sauce for dipping.

4. Enjoy this light and refreshing snack!

Nutrition Facts (per serving):

- Calories: 50
- Total Fat: 1g
- Saturated Fat: 0g
- Cholesterol: 5mg
- Sodium: 30mg
- Total Carbohydrates: 7g
- Dietary Fiber: 1g
- Sugars: 4g
- Protein: 5g

Apple Slices with Almond Butter

Prep Time: 5 mins

Total Time: 5 mins

Servings: 2

Ingredients:

- 1 medium apple, sliced
- 2 tablespoons almond butter

Directions:

1. Slice the apple into wedges.
2. Spread almond butter on apple slices.
3. Serve immediately and enjoy this nutritious and satisfying snack!

Nutrition Facts (per serving):

- Calories: 150
- Total Fat: 9g
- Saturated Fat: 1g

- Cholesterol: 0mg

- Sodium: 0mg

- Total Carbohydrates: 18g

- Dietary Fiber: 4g

- Sugars: 12g

- Protein: 3g

Roasted Chickpeas

Prep Time: 5 mins

Total Time: 30 mins

Servings: 2

Ingredients:

- 1 can (15 oz.) chickpeas, drained and rinsed

- 1 tablespoon olive oil

- 1/2 teaspoon garlic powder

- 1/2 teaspoon paprika

- Salt and pepper to taste

Directions:

1. Preheat oven to 400°F (200°C). Line a baking sheet with parchment paper.

2. Pat dry the chickpeas with a paper towel to remove excess moisture.

3. In a bowl, toss chickpeas with olive oil, garlic powder, paprika, salt, and pepper until evenly coated.

4. Spread chickpeas in a single layer on the prepared baking sheet.

5. Roast in the preheated oven for 20-25 minutes, stirring halfway through, until chickpeas are crispy and golden brown.

6. Remove from oven and let cool for a few minutes before serving.

7. Enjoy these crunchy and flavorful roasted chickpeas!

Nutrition Facts (per serving):

- Calories: 200
- Total Fat: 6g
- Saturated Fat: 1g
- Cholesterol: 0mg
- Sodium: 300mg
- Total Carbohydrates: 30g
- Dietary Fiber: 8g
- Sugars: 3g
- Protein: 9g

DESSERTS RECIPES

Chia Seed Pudding

Prep Time: 5 mins

Total Time: 4 hours 5 mins (includes chilling time)

Servings: 2

Ingredients:

- 1/4 cup chia seeds
- 1 cup unsweetened almond milk
- 1 tablespoon honey or maple syrup
- 1/2 teaspoon vanilla extract
- Fresh berries for topping (optional)

Directions:

1. In a bowl, mix together chia seeds, almond milk, honey or maple syrup, and vanilla extract.
2. Cover and refrigerate for at least 4 hours or overnight, until the mixture thickens and forms a pudding-like consistency.
3. Stir well before serving and top with fresh berries if desired.
4. Enjoy this delicious and nutritious chia seed pudding as a satisfying dessert or snack!

Nutrition Facts (per serving):

- Calories: 150
- Total Fat: 8g
- Saturated Fat: 1g
- Cholesterol: 0mg
- Sodium: 80mg

- Total Carbohydrates: 18g

- Dietary Fiber: 9g

- Sugars: 6g

- Protein: 4g

Baked Apples with Cinnamon

Prep Time: 10 mins

Total Time: 40 mins

Servings: 2

Ingredients:

- 2 apples

- 1 tablespoon melted coconut oil

- 1 teaspoon ground cinnamon

- 1 tablespoon honey or maple syrup

- 2 tablespoons chopped nuts (such as walnuts or almonds)

- Greek yogurt or coconut yogurt for serving (optional)

Directions:

1. Preheat oven to 375°F (190°C). Core the apples and slice off the top to create a well for the filling.

2. In a small bowl, mix together melted coconut oil, ground cinnamon, and honey or maple syrup.

3. Brush the inside of each apple with the cinnamon mixture.

4. Place the apples in a baking dish and bake for 30-35 minutes, until tender.

5. Remove from oven and let cool slightly before serving.

6. Sprinkle chopped nuts over the baked apples and serve with a dollop of Greek yogurt or coconut yogurt if desired.

7. Enjoy these warm and comforting baked apples as a guilt-free dessert!

Nutrition Facts (per serving):

- Calories: 200
- Total Fat: 8g
- Saturated Fat: 4g
- Cholesterol: 0mg
- Sodium: 0mg
- Total Carbohydrates: 30g
- Dietary Fiber: 6g
- Sugars: 20g
- Protein: 2g

Frozen Yogurt Bark

Prep Time: 5 mins

Total Time: 4 hours 5 mins (includes freezing time)

Servings: 4

Ingredients:

- 1 cup Greek yogurt
- 2 tablespoons honey or maple syrup
- 1/2 cup mixed berries (such as strawberries, blueberries, raspberries)
- 2 tablespoons chopped nuts (such as almonds or pistachios)

Directions:

1. Line a baking sheet with parchment paper.

2. In a bowl, mix together Greek yogurt and honey or maple syrup until well combined.

3. Spread the yogurt mixture evenly onto the prepared baking sheet.

4. Sprinkle mixed berries and chopped nuts over the yogurt.

5. Place the baking sheet in the freezer and freeze for at least 4 hours, or until the yogurt bark is firm.

6. Once frozen, break the bark into pieces and serve immediately.

7. Enjoy this refreshing and protein-packed frozen yogurt bark as a healthy dessert or snack!

Nutrition Facts (per serving):

- Calories: 100
- Total Fat: 4g
- Saturated Fat: 1g
- Cholesterol: 0mg
- Sodium: 20mg
- Total Carbohydrates: 14g
- Dietary Fiber: 2g
- Sugars: 10g
- Protein: 5g

Dark Chocolate Avocado Mousse

Prep Time: 10 mins

Total Time: 10 mins

Servings: 2

Ingredients:

- 1 ripe avocado

- 2 tablespoons unsweetened cocoa powder

- 2 tablespoons honey or maple syrup

- 1/2 teaspoon vanilla extract

- Pinch of salt

- Fresh berries for topping (optional)

Directions:

1. Scoop the flesh of the avocado into a blender or food processor.

2. Add cocoa powder, honey or maple syrup, vanilla extract, and a pinch of salt.

3. Blend until smooth and creamy, scraping down the sides of the blender or food processor as needed.

4. Divide the mousse into serving bowls and chill in the refrigerator for at least 30 minutes.

5. Garnish with fresh berries before serving if desired.

6. Enjoy this rich and indulgent dark chocolate avocado mousse as a guilt-free dessert!

Nutrition Facts (per serving):

- Calories: 200

- Total Fat: 10g

- Saturated Fat: 2g

- Cholesterol: 0mg

- Sodium: 5mg

- Total Carbohydrates: 27g

- Dietary Fiber: 7g

- Sugars: 17g

- Protein: 3g

Coconut Date Balls

Prep Time: 10 mins

Total Time: 40 mins

Servings: 10

Ingredients:

- 1 cup pitted dates
- 1 cup unsweetened shredded coconut
- 1/4 cup raw almonds
- 1 tablespoon coconut oil
- 1/2 teaspoon vanilla extract
- Pinch of salt

Directions:

1. Place dates, shredded coconut, almonds, coconut oil, vanilla extract, and a pinch of salt in a food processor.
2. Pulse until the mixture comes together and forms a sticky dough.
3. Roll the dough into small balls using your hands.
4. Place the coconut date balls on a plate or baking sheet lined with parchment paper.
5. Chill in the refrigerator for at least 30 minutes before serving.
6. Enjoy these naturally sweet and satisfying coconut date balls as a nutritious dessert or snack!

Nutrition Facts (per serving):

- Calories: 120
- Total Fat: 6g

- Saturated Fat: 4g

- Cholesterol: 0mg

- Sodium: 10mg

- Total Carbohydrates: 16g

- Dietary Fiber: 3g

- Sugars: 12g

- Protein: 1g

Avocado Chocolate Pudding

Prep Time: 10 mins

Total Time: 10 mins

Servings: 2

Ingredients:

- 1 ripe avocado

- 2 tablespoons unsweetened cocoa powder

- 2 tablespoons honey or maple syrup

- 1/2 teaspoon vanilla extract

- Pinch of salt

- Fresh berries for topping (optional)

Directions:

1. Scoop the flesh of the avocado into a blender or food processor.

2. Add cocoa powder, honey or maple syrup, vanilla extract, and a pinch of salt.

3. Blend until smooth and creamy, scraping down the sides of the blender or food processor as needed.

4. Divide the pudding into serving bowls and chill in the refrigerator for at least 30 minutes.

5. Garnish with fresh berries before serving if desired.

6. Enjoy this rich and creamy avocado chocolate pudding as a guilt-free dessert!

Nutrition Facts (per serving):

- Calories: 180
- Total Fat: 10g
- Saturated Fat: 2g
- Cholesterol: 0mg
- Sodium: 5mg
- Total Carbohydrates: 25g
- Dietary Fiber: 6g
- Sugars: 16g
- Protein: 2g

Berry Chia Seed Parfait

Prep Time: 10 mins

Total Time: 4 hours 10 mins (includes chilling time)

Servings: 2

Ingredients:

- 1 cup mixed berries (such as strawberries, blueberries, raspberries)
- 2 tablespoons chia seeds
- 1 cup unsweetened almond milk
- 1 tablespoon honey or maple syrup

- 1/2 teaspoon vanilla extract
- 2 tablespoons granola for topping (optional)

Directions:

1. In a bowl, mix together chia seeds, almond milk, honey or maple syrup, and vanilla extract.
2. Cover and refrigerate for at least 4 hours or overnight, until the chia pudding thickens.
3. In serving glasses, layer the mixed berries and chia pudding.
4. Repeat the layers until the glasses are filled.
5. Top with granola for some crunch if desired.
6. Chill in the refrigerator for 10 minutes before serving.
7. Enjoy this refreshing and nutritious berry chia seed parfait as a delightful dessert!

Nutrition Facts (per serving):

- Calories: 160
- Total Fat: 6g
- Saturated Fat: 0.5g
- Cholesterol: 0mg
- Sodium: 50mg
- Total Carbohydrates: 25g
- Dietary Fiber: 8g
- Sugars: 13g
- Protein: 4g

Baked Cinnamon Apple Slices

Prep Time: 10 mins

Total Time: 30 mins

Servings: 2

Ingredients:

- 2 apples (such as Granny Smith or Gala)
- 1 tablespoon melted coconut oil
- 1 teaspoon ground cinnamon
- 1 tablespoon honey or maple syrup
- 2 tablespoons chopped walnuts or almonds

Directions:

1. Preheat oven to 375°F (190°C). Line a baking sheet with parchment paper.
2. Core the apples and slice them thinly.
3. In a bowl, toss the apple slices with melted coconut oil, ground cinnamon, and honey or maple syrup until evenly coated.
4. Arrange the apple slices in a single layer on the prepared baking sheet.
5. Sprinkle chopped nuts over the apple slices.
6. Bake for 20-25 minutes, until the apples are tender and lightly browned.
7. Remove from oven and let cool slightly before serving.
8. Enjoy these warm and fragrant baked cinnamon apple slices as a comforting dessert!

Nutrition Facts (per serving):

- Calories: 180
- Total Fat: 9g

- Saturated Fat: 3g

- Cholesterol: 0mg

- Sodium: 0mg

- Total Carbohydrates: 27g

- Dietary Fiber: 5g

- Sugars: 20g

- Protein: 1g

Coconut Yogurt Parfait

Prep Time: 10 mins

Total Time: 10 mins

Servings: 2

Ingredients:

- 1 cup coconut yogurt

- 1/2 cup mixed berries (such as strawberries, blueberries, raspberries)

- 2 tablespoons unsweetened shredded coconut

- 2 tablespoons chopped almonds or pecans

Directions:

1. In serving glasses, layer coconut yogurt, mixed berries, and shredded coconut.

2. Repeat the layers until the glasses are filled.

3. Top with chopped nuts for some crunch.

4. Serve immediately or chill in the refrigerator until ready to serve.

5. Enjoy this creamy and refreshing coconut yogurt parfait as a satisfying dessert!

Nutrition Facts (per serving):

- Calories: 180
- Total Fat: 12g
- Saturated Fat: 6g
- Cholesterol: 0mg
- Sodium: 20mg
- Total Carbohydrates: 16g
- Dietary Fiber: 4g
- Sugars: 10g
- Protein: 3g

Banana Nice Cream

Prep Time: 5 mins

Total Time: 5 mins

Servings: 2

Ingredients:

- 2 ripe bananas, sliced and frozen
- 2 tablespoons unsweetened almond milk or coconut milk
- 1/2 teaspoon vanilla extract
- Toppings of choice: chopped nuts, shredded coconut, dark chocolate chips

Directions:

1. Place frozen banana slices, almond milk or coconut milk, and vanilla extract in a blender or food processor.

2. Blend until smooth and creamy, scraping down the sides of the blender or food processor as needed.

3. Transfer the banana nice cream to serving bowls.

4. Sprinkle with toppings of choice, such as chopped nuts, shredded coconut, or dark chocolate chips.

5. Serve immediately for a soft-serve texture or freeze for 30 minutes for a firmer consistency.

6. Enjoy this guilt-free and delicious banana nice cream as a wholesome dessert!

Nutrition Facts (per serving):

- Calories: 150
- Total Fat: 3g
- Saturated Fat: 1g
- Cholesterol: 0mg
- Sodium: 5mg
- Total Carbohydrates: 33g
- Dietary Fiber: 4g
- Sugars: 18g
- Protein: 2g

Chia Seed Pudding

Prep Time: 5 mins

Total Time: 4 hours 5 mins (includes chilling time)

Servings: 2

Ingredients:

- 1/4 cup chia seeds

- 1 cup unsweetened almond milk
- 1 tablespoon honey or maple syrup
- 1/2 teaspoon vanilla extract
- Fresh berries for topping (optional)

Directions:

1. In a bowl, whisk together chia seeds, almond milk, honey or maple syrup, and vanilla extract.
2. Cover and refrigerate for at least 4 hours or overnight, until the chia pudding thickens.
3. Stir the pudding before serving and divide it into serving bowls.
4. Top with fresh berries if desired.
5. Enjoy this creamy and nutritious chia seed pudding as a guilt-free dessert!

Nutrition Facts (per serving):

- Calories: 150
- Total Fat: 8g
- Saturated Fat: 1g
- Cholesterol: 0mg
- Sodium: 80mg
- Total Carbohydrates: 16g
- Dietary Fiber: 10g
- Sugars: 4g
- Protein: 5g

Baked Cinnamon Banana Chips

Prep Time: 5 mins

Total Time: 2 hours 35 mins

Servings: 2

Ingredients:

- 2 ripe bananas
- 1 tablespoon lemon juice
- 1 teaspoon ground cinnamon

Directions:

1. Preheat oven to 200°F (95°C). Line a baking sheet with parchment paper.
2. Peel the bananas and slice them thinly.
3. Place the banana slices on the prepared baking sheet.
4. Brush the banana slices with lemon juice to prevent browning.
5. Sprinkle ground cinnamon over the banana slices.
6. Bake for 2 to 2.5 hours, flipping the slices halfway through, until they are crispy.
7. Remove from oven and let cool completely before serving.
8. Enjoy these crunchy and naturally sweet baked cinnamon banana chips as a wholesome dessert!

Nutrition Facts (per serving):

- Calories: 120
- Total Fat: 0.5g
- Saturated Fat: 0g
- Cholesterol: 0mg
- Sodium: 0mg
- Total Carbohydrates: 31g

- Dietary Fiber: 4g

- Sugars: 16g

- Protein: 1g

Greek Yogurt with Honey and Walnuts

Prep Time: 5 mins

Total Time: 5 mins

Servings: 2

Ingredients:

- 1 cup plain Greek yogurt

- 2 tablespoons honey

- 2 tablespoons chopped walnuts

Directions:

1. In serving bowls, divide the Greek yogurt.

2. Drizzle honey over the yogurt.

3. Sprinkle chopped walnuts on top.

4. Serve immediately as a simple and satisfying dessert option.

5. Enjoy the creamy texture of Greek yogurt paired with the sweetness of honey and the crunch of walnuts!

Nutrition Facts (per serving):

- Calories: 220

- Total Fat: 11g

- Saturated Fat: 1g

- Cholesterol: 10mg

- Sodium: 40mg

- Total Carbohydrates: 20g

- Dietary Fiber: 1g

- Sugars: 18g

- Protein: 13g

Berry Coconut Popsicles

Prep Time: 10 mins

Total Time: 6 hours 10 mins (includes freezing time)

Servings: 4

Ingredients:

- 1 cup mixed berries (such as strawberries, blueberries, raspberries)

- 1 cup coconut water

- 1 tablespoon honey or maple syrup

Directions:

1. In a blender, combine mixed berries, coconut water, and honey or maple syrup.

2. Blend until smooth.

3. Pour the mixture into popsicle molds.

4. Insert popsicle sticks into the molds.

5. Freeze for at least 6 hours or until completely frozen.

6. Run the molds under warm water to release the popsicles before serving.

7. Enjoy these refreshing and naturally sweet berry coconut popsicles as a delightful treat!

Nutrition Facts (per serving):

- Calories: 40

- Total Fat: 0g

- Saturated Fat: 0g

- Cholesterol: 0mg

- Sodium: 10mg

- Total Carbohydrates: 10g

- Dietary Fiber: 2g

- Sugars: 7g

- Protein: 1g

Baked Apple with Cinnamon

Prep Time: 10 mins

Total Time: 40 mins

Servings: 2

Ingredients:

- 2 apples, cored and halved

- 1 teaspoon cinnamon

- 1 tablespoon honey or maple syrup

- 1 tablespoon chopped walnuts (optional)

Directions:

1. Preheat oven to 375°F (190°C).

2. Place the apple halves in a baking dish, cut side up.

3. Sprinkle cinnamon evenly over the apples.

4. Drizzle honey or maple syrup over the apples.

5. Bake for 30-35 minutes until the apples are tender.

6. Optionally, sprinkle chopped walnuts over the baked apples before serving.

7. Enjoy this warm and comforting dessert that's naturally sweet and full of flavor!

Nutrition Facts (per serving):

- Calories: 120
- Total Fat: 1g
- Saturated Fat: 0g
- Cholesterol: 0mg
- Sodium: 0mg
- Total Carbohydrates: 31g
- Dietary Fiber: 5g
- Sugars: 24g
- Protein: 1g

Avocado Chocolate Mousse

Prep Time: 10 mins

Total Time: 10 mins

Servings: 2

Ingredients:

- 1 ripe avocado
- 2 tablespoons unsweetened cocoa powder
- 2 tablespoons honey or maple syrup
- 1 teaspoon vanilla extract
- Pinch of salt
- Fresh berries for topping (optional)

Directions:

1. In a blender or food processor, combine the avocado, cocoa powder, honey or maple syrup, vanilla extract, and a pinch of salt.

2. Blend until smooth and creamy.

3. Divide the chocolate mousse into serving bowls.

4. Optionally, top with fresh berries before serving.

5. Enjoy this rich and indulgent dessert that's packed with healthy fats and antioxidants!

Nutrition Facts (per serving):

- Calories: 200
- Total Fat: 11g
- Saturated Fat: 2g
- Cholesterol: 0mg
- Sodium: 5mg
- Total Carbohydrates: 28g
- Dietary Fiber: 7g
- Sugars: 18g
- Protein: 3g

Coconut Chia Seed Pudding

Prep Time: 5 mins

Total Time: 4 hours 5 mins (includes chilling time)

Servings: 2

Ingredients:

- 1/4 cup chia seeds
- 1 cup unsweetened coconut milk

- 1 tablespoon honey or maple syrup

- 1/2 teaspoon vanilla extract

- Unsweetened shredded coconut for topping (optional)

Directions:

1. In a bowl, whisk together chia seeds, coconut milk, honey or maple syrup, and vanilla extract.

2. Cover and refrigerate for at least 4 hours or overnight, until the chia pudding thickens.

3. Stir the pudding before serving and divide it into serving bowls.

4. Optionally, sprinkle unsweetened shredded coconut on top before serving.

5. Enjoy this creamy and coco nutty chia seed pudding as a delightful dessert option!

Nutrition Facts (per serving):

- Calories: 180

- Total Fat: 12g

- Saturated Fat: 8g

- Cholesterol: 0mg

- Sodium: 20mg

- Total Carbohydrates: 18g

- Dietary Fiber: 9g

- Sugars: 5g

- Protein: 4g

Frozen Yogurt Bark

Ingredients:

- 2 cups plain Greek yogurt
- 2 tablespoons honey or maple syrup
- 1/2 cup mixed berries (such as strawberries, blueberries, raspberries)
- 1/4 cup chopped nuts (such as almonds, walnuts)
- Unsweetened shredded coconut for topping (optional)

Directions:

1. In a bowl, mix together Greek yogurt and honey or maple syrup.
2. Line a baking sheet with parchment paper.
3. Spread the yogurt mixture evenly on the parchment paper.
4. Sprinkle mixed berries and chopped nuts over the yogurt.
5. Optionally, sprinkle unsweetened shredded coconut on top.
6. Freeze for about 3 hours or until the yogurt bark is firm.
7. Break the frozen yogurt bark into pieces before serving.
8. Enjoy this refreshing and customizable frozen treat as a guilt-free dessert!

Nutrition Facts (per serving):

- Calories: 140
- Total Fat: 6g
- Saturated Fat: 1g
- Cholesterol: 5mg
- Sodium: 25mg

- Total Carbohydrates: 13g

- Dietary Fiber: 2g

- Sugars: 9g

- Protein: 9g

SEAFOOD RECIPES

Grilled Salmon with Lemon and Herbs

Prep Time: 10 mins

Cooking Time: 10 mins

Total Time: 20 mins

Servings: 2

Ingredients:

- 2 salmon fillets
- 1 lemon, sliced
- 2 tablespoons olive oil
- 2 cloves garlic, minced
- 1 tablespoon fresh parsley, chopped
- Salt and pepper to taste

Directions:

1. Preheat grill to medium-high heat.
2. In a small bowl, mix together olive oil, minced garlic, chopped parsley, salt, and pepper.
3. Brush the mixture onto both sides of the salmon fillets.
4. Place lemon slices on top of the salmon.
5. Grill the salmon for about 4-5 minutes per side, or until cooked through and lightly charred.
6. Serve hot with additional lemon wedges if desired.
7. Enjoy this flavorful and nutritious grilled salmon as a delicious seafood option for your fatty liver diet!

Nutritional Information (per serving):

- Calories: 320
- Total Fat: 20g
- Saturated Fat: 3g
- Cholesterol: 90mg
- Sodium: 80mg
- Total Carbohydrates: 3g
- Dietary Fiber: 1g
- Sugars: 1g
- Protein: 30g

Baked Cod with Garlic and Herbs

Prep Time: 10 mins

Cooking Time: 15 mins

Total Time: 25 mins

Servings: 2

Ingredients:

- 2 cod fillets
- 2 cloves garlic, minced
- 2 tablespoons olive oil
- 1 tablespoon fresh lemon juice
- 1 teaspoon dried thyme
- Salt and pepper to taste
- Fresh parsley for garnish

Directions:

1. Preheat oven to 400°F (200°C).
2. Place the cod fillets in a baking dish.

3. In a small bowl, mix together minced garlic, olive oil, lemon juice, dried thyme, salt, and pepper.

4. Pour the mixture over the cod fillets, ensuring they are evenly coated.

5. Bake in the preheated oven for 12-15 minutes, or until the cod is opaque and flakes easily with a fork.

6. Garnish with fresh parsley before serving.

7. Enjoy this tender and flavorful baked cod as a healthy seafood option for your fatty liver diet!

Nutritional Information (per serving):

- Calories: 220
- Total Fat: 10g
- Saturated Fat: 2g
- Cholesterol: 60mg
- Sodium: 150mg
- Total Carbohydrates: 2g
- Dietary Fiber: 0g
- Sugars: 0g
- Protein: 30g

Shrimp Stir-Fry

Prep Time: 15 mins

Cooking Time: 10 mins

Total Time: 25 mins

Servings: 2

Ingredients:

- 1/2 lb shrimp, peeled and deveined
- 2 cups mixed vegetables (such as bell peppers, broccoli, carrots)
- 2 cloves garlic, minced
- 1 tablespoon olive oil
- 2 tablespoons low-sodium soy sauce
- 1 teaspoon sesame oil
- 1 teaspoon honey or maple syrup
- Cooked brown rice for serving

Directions:

1. Heat olive oil in a skillet over medium-high heat.
2. Add minced garlic and cook until fragrant, about 1 minute.
3. Add shrimp to the skillet and cook for 2-3 minutes, until pink and cooked through.
4. Add mixed vegetables to the skillet and stir-fry for 3-4 minutes, until tender-crisp.
5. In a small bowl, mix together low-sodium soy sauce, sesame oil, and honey or maple syrup.
6. Pour the sauce over the shrimp and vegetables, and toss to coat evenly.
7. Serve hot over cooked brown rice.
8. Enjoy this quick and delicious shrimp stir-fry as a nutritious seafood option for your fatty liver diet!

Nutritional Information (per serving without rice):

- Calories: 180
- Total Fat: 7g
- Saturated Fat: 1g

- Cholesterol: 120mg

- Sodium: 400mg

- Total Carbohydrates: 10g

- Dietary Fiber: 3g

- Sugars: 5g

- Protein: 20g

Tuna Salad Lettuce Wraps

Prep Time: 10 mins

Total Time: 10 mins

Servings: 2

Ingredients:

- 1 can (5 oz) tuna, drained

- 2 tablespoons plain Greek yogurt

- 1 tablespoon Dijon mustard

- 1 celery stalk, finely chopped

- 1/4 red onion, finely chopped

- Salt and pepper to taste

- 4 large lettuce leaves

Directions:

1. In a bowl, combine drained tuna, Greek yogurt, Dijon mustard, chopped celery, and chopped red onion.

2. Mix well until all ingredients are evenly incorporated.

3. Season with salt and pepper to taste.

4. Divide the tuna salad mixture among the lettuce leaves.

5. Wrap the lettuce leaves around the tuna salad, forming lettuce wraps.

6. Serve immediately or refrigerate until ready to eat.

7. Enjoy these light and refreshing tuna salad lettuce wraps as a healthy seafood snack or meal option for your fatty liver diet!

Nutritional Information (per serving):

- Calories: 120
- Total Fat: 3g
- Saturated Fat: 0.5g
- Cholesterol: 25mg
- Sodium: 300mg
- Total Carbohydrates: 4g
- Dietary Fiber: 1g
- Sugars: 1g
- Protein: 20g

Baked Lemon Garlic Tilapia

Prep Time: 10 mins

Cooking Time: 15 mins

Total Time: 25 mins

Servings: 2

Ingredients:

- 2 tilapia fillets
- 2 cloves garlic, minced
- 1 lemon, sliced
- 2 tablespoons olive oil

- 1 teaspoon dried oregano
- Salt and pepper to taste
- Fresh parsley for garnish

Directions:

1. Preheat oven to 400°F (200°C).
2. Place tilapia fillets in a baking dish.
3. In a small bowl, whisk together minced garlic, olive oil, dried oregano, salt, and pepper.
4. Pour the mixture over the tilapia fillets, ensuring they are evenly coated.
5. Place lemon slices on top of the fillets.
6. Bake in the preheated oven for 12-15 minutes, or until the fish is opaque and flakes easily with a fork.
7. Garnish with fresh parsley before serving.
8. Enjoy this light and flavorful baked tilapia as a healthy seafood option for your fatty liver diet!

Nutritional Information (per serving):

- Calories: 200
- Total Fat: 10g
- Saturated Fat: 1.5g
- Cholesterol: 60mg
- Sodium: 80mg
- Total Carbohydrates: 3g
- Dietary Fiber: 1g
- Sugars: 1g
- Protein: 25g

Grilled Shrimp Skewers

Prep Time: 15 mins

Cooking Time: 10 mins

Total Time: 25 mins

Servings: 2

Ingredients:

- 1/2 lb. large shrimp, peeled and deveined
- 1 bell pepper, cut into chunks
- 1 red onion, cut into chunks
- 2 tablespoons olive oil
- 2 cloves garlic, minced
- 1 teaspoon paprika
- Salt and pepper to taste
- Wooden skewers, soaked in water for 30 minutes

Directions:

1. Preheat grill to medium-high heat.
2. In a bowl, combine olive oil, minced garlic, paprika, salt, and pepper.
3. Thread shrimp, bell pepper chunks, and red onion chunks onto the soaked wooden skewers.
4. Brush the skewers with the olive oil mixture.
5. Grill the skewers for 2-3 minutes per side, or until the shrimp are pink and cooked through.
6. Serve hot with your favorite dipping sauce or over a bed of quinoa or brown rice.

7. Enjoy these delicious and colorful grilled shrimp skewers as a nutritious seafood option for your fatty liver diet!

Nutritional Information (per serving):

- Calories: 180
- Total Fat: 10g
- Saturated Fat: 1.5g
- Cholesterol: 120mg
- Sodium: 300mg
- Total Carbohydrates: 8g
- Dietary Fiber: 2g
- Sugars: 3g
- Protein: 15g

Salmon Salad with Avocado Dressing

Prep Time: 15 mins

Cooking Time: 10 mins

Total Time: 25 mins

Servings: 2

Ingredients:

- 2 salmon fillets
- 4 cups mixed salad greens
- 1 avocado, diced
- 1/4 cup cherry tomatoes, halved
- 1/4 cup cucumber, sliced
- 2 tablespoons olive oil
- 1 tablespoon lemon juice

- 1 teaspoon Dijon mustard
- Salt and pepper to taste

Directions:

1. Season salmon fillets with salt and pepper, then grill or bake until cooked through.
2. In a large bowl, combine mixed salad greens, diced avocado, cherry tomatoes, and cucumber slices.
3. In a small bowl, whisk together olive oil, lemon juice, Dijon mustard, salt, and pepper to make the dressing.
4. Pour the dressing over the salad and toss to coat evenly.
5. Divide the salad onto plates and top with grilled salmon fillets.
6. Serve immediately and enjoy this fresh and flavorful salmon salad as a healthy seafood option for your fatty liver diet!

Nutritional Information (per serving):

- Calories: 320
- Total Fat: 22g
- Saturated Fat: 3.5g
- Cholesterol: 80mg
- Sodium: 150mg
- Total Carbohydrates: 10g
- Dietary Fiber: 6g
- Sugars: 2g
- Protein: 25g

Baked Lemon Herb Mahi Mahi

Prep Time: 10 mins

Cooking Time: 15 mins

Total Time: 25 mins

Servings: 2

Ingredients:

- 2 mahi mahi fillets
- 1 lemon, sliced
- 2 tablespoons olive oil
- 2 cloves garlic, minced
- 1 teaspoon dried basil
- Salt and pepper to taste
- Fresh parsley for garnish

Directions:

1. Preheat oven to 400°F (200°C).
2. Place Mahi Mahi fillets in a baking dish.
3. In a small bowl, whisk together olive oil, minced garlic, dried basil, salt, and pepper.
4. Pour the mixture over the Mahi Mahi fillets, ensuring they are evenly coated.
5. Place lemon slices on top of the fillets.
6. Bake in the preheated oven for 12-15 minutes, or until the fish is opaque and flakes easily with a fork.
7. Garnish with fresh parsley before serving.
8. Enjoy this light and flavorful baked Mahi Mahi as a nutritious seafood option for your fatty liver diet!

Nutritional Information (per serving):

- Calories: 220

- Total Fat: 12g

- Saturated Fat: 1.5g

- Cholesterol: 100mg

- Sodium: 120mg

- Total Carbohydrates: 2g

- Dietary Fiber: 1g

- Sugars: 0g

- Protein: 25g

Coconut Shrimp with Mango Salsa

Prep Time: 20 mins

Cooking Time: 10 mins

Total Time: 30 mins

Servings: 2

Ingredients:

- 1/2 lb. large shrimp, peeled and deveined

- 1/2 cup shredded coconut

- 1/4 cup panko breadcrumbs

- 1 egg, beaten

- Salt and pepper to taste

- Olive oil cooking spray

Mango Salsa:

- 1 ripe mango, diced

- 1/4 cup red onion, finely chopped

- 1/4 cup red bell pepper, diced

- 2 tablespoons fresh cilantro, chopped
- 1 tablespoon lime juice
- Salt and pepper to taste

Directions:

1. Preheat oven to 400°F (200°C).
2. In one bowl, combine shredded coconut and panko breadcrumbs.
3. In another bowl, beat the egg and season with salt and pepper.
4. Dip each shrimp into the beaten egg, then coat with the coconut breadcrumb mixture.
5. Place the coated shrimp on a baking sheet lined with parchment paper.
6. Lightly spray the shrimp with olive oil cooking spray.
7. Bake in the preheated oven for 8-10 minutes, or until the shrimp are golden brown and cooked through.
8. While the shrimp are baking, prepare the mango salsa by combining diced mango, red onion, red bell pepper, cilantro, lime juice, salt, and pepper in a bowl.
9. Serve the coconut shrimp hot with mango salsa on the side.
10. Enjoy this tropical-inspired dish as a delicious and healthy seafood option for your fatty liver diet!

Nutritional Information (per serving, including salsa):

- Calories: 280
- Total Fat: 12g
- Saturated Fat: 6g
- Cholesterol: 200mg

- Sodium: 250mg

- Total Carbohydrates: 20g

- Dietary Fiber: 3g

- Sugars: 12g

- Protein: 22g

Grilled Lemon Herb Salmon

Prep Time: 10 mins

Cooking Time: 10 mins

Total Time: 20 mins

Servings: 2

Ingredients:

- 2 salmon fillets

- 2 tablespoons olive oil

- 1 lemon, juiced and zested

- 2 cloves garlic, minced

- 1 teaspoon dried thyme

- 1 teaspoon dried rosemary

- Salt and pepper to taste

- Fresh parsley for garnish

Directions:

1. Preheat grill to medium-high heat.

2. In a small bowl, whisk together olive oil, lemon juice, lemon zest, minced garlic, dried thyme, dried rosemary, salt, and pepper.

3. Place salmon fillets on a plate and brush both sides with the lemon herb mixture.

4. Grill the salmon fillets for 4-5 minutes per side, or until cooked through and flaky.

5. Garnish with fresh parsley before serving.

6. Enjoy this flavorful grilled lemon herb salmon as a healthy seafood option for your fatty liver diet!

Nutritional Information (per serving):

- Calories: 280

- Total Fat: 18g

- Saturated Fat: 3g

- Cholesterol: 80mg

- Sodium: 70mg

- Total Carbohydrates: 2g

- Dietary Fiber: 1g

- Sugars: 0g

- Protein: 26g

Baked Cod with Tomatoes and Olives

Prep Time: 15 mins

Cooking Time: 20 mins

Total Time: 35 mins

Servings: 2

Ingredients:

- 2 cod fillets

- 1 cup cherry tomatoes, halved

- 1/4 cup pitted kalamata olives, sliced

- 2 tablespoons olive oil

- 2 cloves garlic, minced

- 1 tablespoon fresh basil, chopped

- Salt and pepper to taste

- Lemon wedges for serving

Directions:

1. Preheat oven to 400°F (200°C).

2. Place cod fillets in a baking dish.

3. In a bowl, combine cherry tomatoes, sliced Kalamata olives, minced garlic, chopped basil, olive oil, salt, and pepper.

4. Spoon the tomato and olive mixture over the cod fillets.

5. Bake in the preheated oven for 15-20 minutes, or until the fish is opaque and flakes easily with a fork.

6. Serve hot with lemon wedges on the side.

7. Enjoy this Mediterranean-inspired baked cod with tomatoes and olives as a nutritious seafood option for your fatty liver diet!

Nutritional Information (per serving):

- Calories: 220

- Total Fat: 12g

- Saturated Fat: 2g

- Cholesterol: 60mg

- Sodium: 350mg

- Total Carbohydrates: 5g

- Dietary Fiber: 2g

- Sugars: 2g

- Protein: 25g

Shrimp Stir-Fry with Vegetables

Prep Time: 15 mins

Cooking Time: 10 mins

Total Time: 25 mins

Servings: 2

Ingredients:

- 1/2 lb. large shrimp, peeled and deveined
- 2 cups mixed vegetables (bell peppers, broccoli, snap peas, carrots)
- 2 cloves garlic, minced
- 1 tablespoon ginger, minced
- 2 tablespoons low-sodium soy sauce
- 1 tablespoon sesame oil
- 1 teaspoon honey
- 1 tablespoon olive oil
- Sesame seeds for garnish
- Cooked brown rice for serving

Directions:

1. Heat olive oil in a large skillet or wok over medium-high heat.
2. Add minced garlic and ginger to the skillet and sauté for 1 minute.
3. Add shrimp to the skillet and cook until pink and opaque, about 2-3 minutes per side. Remove shrimp from the skillet and set aside.

4. In the same skillet, add mixed vegetables and stir-fry until tender-crisp, about 3-4 minutes.

5. Return the cooked shrimp to the skillet with the vegetables.

6. In a small bowl, whisk together low-sodium soy sauce, sesame oil, and honey. Pour the sauce over the shrimp and vegetables, stirring to combine.

7. Cook for an additional 1-2 minutes, until everything is heated through.

8. Serve hot over cooked brown rice, garnished with sesame seeds.

9. Enjoy this delicious shrimp stir-fry with vegetables as a flavorful seafood option for your fatty liver diet!

Nutritional Information (per serving, excluding rice):

- Calories: 220
- Total Fat: 10g
- Saturated Fat: 1.5g
- Cholesterol: 150mg
- Sodium: 500mg
- Total Carbohydrates: 10g
- Dietary Fiber: 3g
- Sugars: 5g
- Protein: 25g

Tuna Salad Lettuce Wraps

Prep Time: 10 mins

Total Time: 10 mins

Servings: 2

Ingredients:

- 1 can (5 oz.) tuna in water, drained
- 2 tablespoons Greek yogurt
- 1 tablespoon lemon juice
- 1/4 cup celery, diced
- 1/4 cup red onion, diced
- 1 tablespoon fresh parsley, chopped
- Salt and pepper to taste
- Lettuce leaves for wrapping

Directions:

1. In a bowl, combine drained tuna, Greek yogurt, lemon juice, diced celery, diced red onion, chopped parsley, salt, and pepper.
2. Mix well until all ingredients are combined.
3. Spoon the tuna salad mixture onto lettuce leaves.
4. Wrap the lettuce leaves around the tuna salad mixture to form lettuce wraps.
5. Serve immediately and enjoy these light and refreshing tuna salad lettuce wraps as a healthy seafood option for your fatty liver diet!

Nutritional Information (per serving, 2 lettuce wraps):

- Calories: 100
- Total Fat: 2g
- Saturated Fat: 0.5g
- Cholesterol: 25mg
- Sodium: 300mg
- Total Carbohydrates: 4g

- Dietary Fiber: 1g

- Sugars: 1g

- Protein: 16g

Baked Halibut with Lemon Garlic Butter

Prep Time: 10 mins

Cooking Time: 15 mins

Total Time: 25 mins

Servings: 2

Ingredients:

- 2 halibut fillets

- 2 tablespoons unsalted butter, melted

- 2 cloves garlic, minced

- 1 tablespoon fresh lemon juice

- 1 teaspoon lemon zest

- Salt and pepper to taste

- Fresh parsley for garnish

Directions:

1. Preheat oven to 400°F (200°C).

2. Place halibut fillets on a baking sheet lined with parchment paper.

3. In a small bowl, combine melted unsalted butter, minced garlic, fresh lemon juice, lemon zest, salt, and pepper.

4. Brush the lemon garlic butter mixture over the halibut fillets.

5. Bake in the preheated oven for 12-15 minutes, or until the fish is opaque and flakes easily with a fork.

6. Garnish with fresh parsley before serving.

7. Enjoy this simple and delicious baked halibut with lemon garlic butter as a nutritious seafood option for your fatty liver diet!

Nutritional Information (per serving):

- Calories: 250
- Total Fat: 12g
- Saturated Fat: 5g
- Cholesterol: 80mg
- Sodium: 300mg
- Total Carbohydrates: 1g
- Dietary Fiber: 0g
- Sugars: 0g
- Protein: 35g

Lemon Garlic Shrimp

Prep Time: 10 mins

Cooking Time: 5 mins

Total Time: 15 mins

Servings: 2

Ingredients:

- 1 lb. large shrimp, peeled and deveined
- 2 tablespoons olive oil
- 4 cloves garlic, minced
- 1 tablespoon lemon juice
- 1 teaspoon lemon zest
- Salt and pepper to taste
- Fresh parsley for garnish

Directions:

1. In a large skillet, heat olive oil over medium heat.

2. Add minced garlic to the skillet and sauté for 1 minute until fragrant.

3. Add shrimp to the skillet and cook for 2-3 minutes on each side until pink and opaque.

4. Stir in lemon juice and lemon zest. Season with salt and pepper to taste.

5. Cook for an additional minute, stirring occasionally.

6. Garnish with fresh parsley before serving.

7. Enjoy this flavorful lemon garlic shrimp as a quick and healthy seafood option for your fatty liver diet!

Nutritional Information (per serving):

- Calories: 250
- Total Fat: 14g
- Saturated Fat: 2g
- Cholesterol: 300mg
- Sodium: 450mg
- Total Carbohydrates: 2g
- Dietary Fiber: 0g
- Sugars: 0g
- Protein: 28g

Baked Salmon with Dill

Prep Time: 10 mins

Cooking Time: 15 mins

Total Time: 25 mins

Servings: 2

Ingredients:

- 2 salmon fillets
- 1 tablespoon olive oil
- 2 tablespoons fresh dill, chopped
- 1 tablespoon lemon juice
- Salt and pepper to taste
- Lemon wedges for serving

Directions:

1. Preheat oven to 400°F (200°C).
2. Place salmon fillets on a baking sheet lined with parchment paper.
3. Drizzle olive oil over the salmon fillets and sprinkle with chopped fresh dill.
4. Squeeze lemon juice over the salmon and season with salt and pepper to taste.
5. Bake in the preheated oven for 12-15 minutes, or until the salmon is cooked through and flakes easily with a fork.
6. Serve hot with lemon wedges on the side.
7. Enjoy this simple and delicious baked salmon with dill as a nutritious seafood option for your fatty liver diet!

Nutritional Information (per serving):

- Calories: 280
- Total Fat: 18g
- Saturated Fat: 3g

- Cholesterol: 80mg

- Sodium: 70mg

- Total Carbohydrates: 2g

- Dietary Fiber: 1g

- Sugars: 0g

- Protein: 26g

Grilled Tilapia with Mango Salsa

Prep Time: 15 mins

Cooking Time: 10 mins

Total Time: 25 mins

Servings: 2

Ingredients:

- 2 tilapia fillets

- 1 tablespoon olive oil

- 1 teaspoon paprika

- 1/2 teaspoon ground cumin

- Salt and pepper to taste

- Mango Salsa:

  - 1 ripe mango, diced

  - 1/4 cup red onion, finely chopped

  - 1/4 cup red bell pepper, diced

  - 2 tablespoons fresh cilantro, chopped

  - 1 tablespoon lime juice

  - Salt and pepper to taste

Directions:

1. Preheat grill to medium-high heat.

2. Brush tilapia fillets with olive oil and season with paprika, ground cumin, salt, and pepper.

3. Grill the tilapia fillets for 3-4 minutes per side, or until cooked through and opaque.

4. In a bowl, combine diced mango, finely chopped red onion, diced red bell pepper, chopped fresh cilantro, lime juice, salt, and pepper to make the mango salsa.

5. Serve grilled tilapia topped with mango salsa.

6. Enjoy this vibrant and flavorful grilled tilapia with mango salsa as a delicious seafood option for your fatty liver diet!

Nutritional Information (per serving):

- Calories: 230

- Total Fat: 8g

- Saturated Fat: 1g

- Cholesterol: 60mg

- Sodium: 120mg

- Total Carbohydrates: 16g

- Dietary Fiber: 2g

- Sugars: 11g

- Protein: 24g

Baked Mahi-Mahi with Herb Crust

Prep Time: 15 mins

Cooking Time: 20 mins

Total Time: 35 mins

Servings: 2

Ingredients:

- 2 mahi-mahi fillets

- 2 tablespoons olive oil

- 2 tablespoons fresh parsley, chopped

- 1 tablespoon fresh basil, chopped

- 1 tablespoon fresh thyme, chopped

- 2 cloves garlic, minced

- Salt and pepper to taste

- Lemon wedges for serving

Directions:

1. Preheat oven to 400°F (200°C).

2. Place mahi-mahi fillets on a baking sheet lined with parchment paper.

3. In a bowl, combine olive oil, chopped fresh parsley, chopped fresh basil, chopped fresh thyme, minced garlic, salt, and pepper to make the herb crust.

4. Spread the herb crust evenly over the mahi-mahi fillets, pressing lightly to adhere.

5. Bake in the preheated oven for 15-20 minutes, or until the fish is opaque and flakes easily with a fork.

6. Serve hot with lemon wedges on the side.

7. Enjoy this flavorful baked mahi-mahi with herb crust as a healthy seafood option for your fatty liver diet!

Nutritional Information (per serving):

- Calories: 260
- Total Fat: 14g
- Saturated Fat: 2g
- Cholesterol: 120mg
- Sodium: 200mg
- Total Carbohydrates: 2g
- Dietary Fiber: 1g
- Sugars: 0g
- Protein: 30g

BEVERAGES RECIPES

Turmeric Ginger Tea

Prep Time: 5 mins

Cooking Time: 10 mins

Total Time: 15 mins

Servings: 2

Ingredients:

- 2 cups water
- 1 teaspoon turmeric powder
- 1 teaspoon grated fresh ginger
- 1 tablespoon honey (optional)
- Lemon slices for garnish (optional)

Directions:

1. In a small saucepan, bring water to a boil.
2. Add turmeric powder and grated ginger to the boiling water.
3. Reduce heat to low and let the mixture simmer for 8-10 minutes.
4. Remove from heat and strain the tea into cups.
5. Stir in honey, if desired, and garnish with lemon slices.
6. Serve hot and enjoy the soothing and detoxifying benefits of turmeric ginger tea for your fatty liver diet!

Nutritional Information (per serving):

- Calories: 15
- Total Fat: 0g
- Saturated Fat: 0g

- Cholesterol: 0mg

- Sodium: 5mg

- Total Carbohydrates: 4g

- Dietary Fiber: 0g

- Sugars: 3g

- Protein: 0g

Cucumber Mint Cooler

Prep Time: 10 mins

Total Time: 10 mins

Servings: 2

Ingredients:

- 1 large cucumber, peeled and chopped

- 1/4 cup fresh mint leaves

- 2 cups water

- 1 tablespoon lemon juice

- Ice cubes

- Cucumber slices and mint sprigs for garnish

Directions:

1. In a blender, combine chopped cucumber, fresh mint leaves, water, and lemon juice.

2. Blend until smooth.

3. Strain the mixture to remove any pulp.

4. Pour the cucumber mint juice into glasses filled with ice cubes.

5. Garnish with cucumber slices and mint sprigs.

6. Serve chilled and enjoy this refreshing cucumber mint cooler as a hydrating beverage for your fatty liver diet!

Nutritional Information (per serving):

- Calories: 10
- Total Fat: 0g
- Saturated Fat: 0g
- Cholesterol: 0mg
- Sodium: 5mg
- Total Carbohydrates: 3g
- Dietary Fiber: 1g
- Sugars: 1g
- Protein: 0g

Berry Blast Smoothie

Prep Time: 5 mins

Total Time: 5 mins

Servings: 2

Ingredients:

- 1 cup mixed berries (such as strawberries, blueberries, raspberries)
- 1/2 cup plain Greek yogurt
- 1/2 cup almond milk
- 1 tablespoon chia seeds
- 1 tablespoon honey (optional)
- Ice cubes

Directions:

1. In a blender, combine mixed berries, Greek yogurt, almond milk, chia seeds, and honey.

2. Blend until smooth and creamy.

3. Add ice cubes and blend again until well combined.

4. Pour the berry smoothie into glasses and serve immediately.

5. Enjoy this antioxidant-rich berry blast smoothie as a delicious and nutritious beverage for your fatty liver diet!

Nutritional Information (per serving):

- Calories: 120

- Total Fat: 3g

- Saturated Fat: 0g

- Cholesterol: 2mg

- Sodium: 50mg

- Total Carbohydrates: 18g

- Dietary Fiber: 6g

- Sugars: 10g

- Protein: 8g

Green Detox Juice

Prep Time: 10 mins

Total Time: 10 mins

Servings: 2

Ingredients:

- 2 cups spinach leaves

- 1 cucumber, peeled and chopped

- 1 green apple, cored and chopped

- 1/2 lemon, peeled
- 1-inch piece of ginger, peeled
- 1 cup water
- Ice cubes

Directions:

1. In a juicer, process spinach leaves, chopped cucumber, chopped green apple, peeled lemon, and peeled ginger.
2. Add water to the juicer and continue to process until all ingredients are juiced.
3. Strain the juice to remove any pulp.
4. Pour the green detox juice into glasses filled with ice cubes.
5. Serve chilled and enjoy this refreshing and nutrient-packed green juice as a cleansing beverage for your fatty liver diet!

Nutritional Information (per serving):

- Calories: 70
- Total Fat: 0g
- Saturated Fat: 0g
- Cholesterol: 0mg
- Sodium: 20mg
- Total Carbohydrates: 18g
- Dietary Fiber: 4g
- Sugars: 10g
- Protein: 2g

Ginger Lemon Detox Water

Prep Time: 5 mins

Total Time: 5 mins

Servings: 2

Ingredients:

- 2 cups filtered water
- 1 tablespoon grated ginger
- 1 lemon, sliced
- Fresh mint leaves for garnish (optional)
- Ice cubes

Directions:

1. In a pitcher, combine filtered water and grated ginger.
2. Add lemon slices to the pitcher.
3. Refrigerate for at least 1 hour to allow the flavors to infuse.
4. Serve chilled over ice cubes, garnished with fresh mint leaves if desired.
5. Enjoy this refreshing ginger lemon detox water as a hydrating beverage for your fatty liver diet!

Nutritional Information (per serving):

- Calories: 0
- Total Fat: 0g
- Saturated Fat: 0g
- Cholesterol: 0mg
- Sodium: 10mg
- Total Carbohydrates: 0g
- Dietary Fiber: 0g
- Sugars: 0g

- Protein: 0g

Green Tea with Mint

Prep Time: 5 mins

Cooking Time: 5 mins

Total Time: 10 mins

Servings: 2

Ingredients:

- 2 cups water
- 2 green tea bags
- 1 tablespoon fresh mint leaves, chopped
- Honey or stevia to taste (optional)
- Lemon slices for garnish (optional)

Directions:

1. In a saucepan, bring water to a boil.
2. Remove from heat and add green tea bags and chopped mint leaves.
3. Let the tea steep for 3-5 minutes.
4. Remove the tea bags and strain the tea to remove the mint leaves.
5. Add honey or stevia to taste, if desired.
6. Pour the green tea into cups and garnish with lemon slices.
7. Serve hot and enjoy the refreshing flavor of green tea with mint for your fatty liver diet!

Nutritional Information (per serving):

- Calories: 0
- Total Fat: 0g

- Saturated Fat: 0g

- Cholesterol: 0mg

- Sodium: 10mg

- Total Carbohydrates: 0g

- Dietary Fiber: 0g

- Sugars: 0g

- Protein: 0g

Golden Milk Latte

Prep Time: 5 mins

Cooking Time: 10 mins

Total Time: 15 mins

Servings: 2

Ingredients:

- 2 cups unsweetened almond milk

- 1 teaspoon ground turmeric

- 1/2 teaspoon ground cinnamon

- 1/4 teaspoon ground ginger

- Pinch of black pepper

- 1 tablespoon honey or maple syrup (optional)

- 1 teaspoon coconut oil (optional)

Directions:

1. In a saucepan, heat almond milk over medium heat until warm but not boiling.

2. Whisk in ground turmeric, ground cinnamon, ground ginger, and black pepper.

3. Stir in honey or maple syrup and coconut oil, if using.

4. Continue to heat for another 2-3 minutes, stirring occasionally.

5. Remove from heat and pour the golden milk latte into cups.

6. Serve warm and enjoy the comforting and anti-inflammatory benefits of golden milk latte for your fatty liver diet!

Nutritional Information (per serving):

- Calories: 50

- Total Fat: 2g

- Saturated Fat: 0g

- Cholesterol: 0mg

- Sodium: 180mg

- Total Carbohydrates: 8g

- Dietary Fiber: 1g

- Sugars: 6g

- Protein: 1g

Berry Hibiscus Iced Tea

Prep Time: 5 mins

Cooking Time: 5 mins

Total Time: 10 mins

Servings: 2

Ingredients:

- 2 cups water

- 2 hibiscus tea bags

- 1/2 cup mixed berries (such as strawberries, blueberries, raspberries)

- Honey or stevia to taste (optional)
- Lemon slices for garnish (optional)
- Ice cubes

Directions:

1. In a saucepan, bring water to a boil.
2. Remove from heat and add hibiscus tea bags.
3. Let the tea bags steep for 5 minutes.
4. Remove the tea bags and allow the tea to cool to room temperature.
5. In a glass pitcher, muddle the mixed berries to release their juices.
6. Pour the cooled hibiscus tea into the pitcher with the muddled berries.
7. Stir in honey or stevia to taste, if desired.
8. Refrigerate for at least 1 hour to chill the tea.
9. Serve over ice cubes, garnished with lemon slices if desired.
10. Enjoy this refreshing berry hibiscus iced tea as a flavorful beverage for your fatty liver diet!

Nutritional Information (per serving):

- Calories: 20
- Total Fat: 0g
- Saturated Fat: 0g
- Cholesterol: 0mg
- Sodium: 10mg
- Total Carbohydrates: 5g
- Dietary Fiber: 1g

- Sugars: 3g

- Protein: 0g

Minty Cucumber Infused Water

Prep Time: 5 mins

Total Time: 5 mins

Servings: 2

Ingredients:

- 4 cups filtered water

- 1 cucumber, thinly sliced

- 10-12 fresh mint leaves

- Ice cubes

Directions:

1. In a pitcher, combine filtered water, sliced cucumber, and fresh mint leaves.

2. Stir well to mix the ingredients.

3. Refrigerate for at least 1 hour to allow the flavors to infuse.

4. Serve chilled over ice cubes.

5. Enjoy this refreshing minty cucumber infused water as a hydrating beverage for your fatty liver diet!

Nutritional Information (per serving):

- Calories: 0

- Total Fat: 0g

- Saturated Fat: 0g

- Cholesterol: 0mg

- Sodium: 0mg

- Total Carbohydrates: 0g

- Dietary Fiber: 0g

- Sugars: 0g

- Protein: 0g

Apple Cider Vinegar Detox Drink

Prep Time: 5 mins

Total Time: 5 mins

Servings: 1

Ingredients:

- 1 cup filtered water

- 2 tablespoons raw apple cider vinegar

- 1 tablespoon fresh lemon juice

- 1 teaspoon honey or maple syrup (optional)

- Pinch of ground cinnamon (optional)

- Ice cubes

Directions:

1. In a glass, combine filtered water, raw apple cider vinegar, and fresh lemon juice.

2. Stir in honey or maple syrup and ground cinnamon, if desired.

3. Add ice cubes to the glass.

4. Stir well to mix all the ingredients.

5. Enjoy this apple cider vinegar detox drink as a cleansing beverage for your fatty liver diet!

Nutritional Information (per serving):

- Calories: 15

- Total Fat: 0g

- Saturated Fat: 0g

- Cholesterol: 0mg

- Sodium: 10mg

- Total Carbohydrates: 4g

- Dietary Fiber: 0g

- Sugars: 3g

- Protein: 0g

Turmeric Golden Milk

Prep Time: 5 mins

Cooking Time: 5 mins

Total Time: 10 mins

Servings: 2

Ingredients:

- 2 cups unsweetened almond milk

- 1 teaspoon ground turmeric

- 1/2 teaspoon ground cinnamon

- 1/4 teaspoon ground ginger

- Pinch of black pepper

- 1 tablespoon honey or maple syrup (optional)

- 1 teaspoon coconut oil (optional)

Directions:

1. In a saucepan, heat almond milk over medium heat until warm but not boiling.

2. Whisk in ground turmeric, ground cinnamon, ground ginger, and black pepper.

3. Stir in honey or maple syrup and coconut oil, if using.

4. Continue to heat for another 2-3 minutes, stirring occasionally.

5. Remove from heat and pour the turmeric golden milk into cups.

6. Serve warm and enjoy the anti-inflammatory benefits of turmeric golden milk for your fatty liver diet!

Nutritional Information (per serving):

- Calories: 50

- Total Fat: 2g

- Saturated Fat: 0g

- Cholesterol: 0mg

- Sodium: 180mg

- Total Carbohydrates: 8g

- Dietary Fiber: 1g

- Sugars: 6g

- Protein: 1g

Berry Blast Smoothie

Prep Time: 5 mins

Total Time: 5 mins

Servings: 2

Ingredients:

- 1 cup mixed berries (such as strawberries, blueberries, raspberries)

- 1 ripe banana

- 1 cup unsweetened almond milk
- 1 tablespoon chia seeds
- Ice cubes

Directions:

1. In a blender, combine mixed berries, ripe banana, unsweetened almond milk, and chia seeds.
2. Blend until smooth and creamy.
3. Add ice cubes to achieve desired consistency and blend again.
4. Pour the berry blast smoothie into glasses.
5. Serve immediately and enjoy this nutritious and delicious smoothie as a satisfying beverage for your fatty liver diet!

Nutritional Information (per serving):

- Calories: 120
- Total Fat: 3g
- Saturated Fat: 0g
- Cholesterol: 0mg
- Sodium: 80mg
- Total Carbohydrates: 22g
- Dietary Fiber: 7g
- Sugars: 11g
- Protein: 3g

Detoxifying Green Tea

Prep Time: 2 mins

Total Time: 5 mins

Servings: 1

Ingredients:

- 1 green tea bag
- 1 cup hot water
- 1 tablespoon fresh lemon juice
- 1 teaspoon honey (optional)
- Ice cubes

Directions:

1. Place the green tea bag in a cup and pour hot water over it.
2. Let it steep for 3-5 minutes.
3. Remove the tea bag and allow the green tea to cool slightly.
4. Stir in fresh lemon juice and honey, if using.
5. Add ice cubes to chill the tea.
6. Stir well and enjoy this refreshing detoxifying green tea as part of your fatty liver diet!

Nutritional Information (per serving):

- Calories: 5
- Total Fat: 0g
- Saturated Fat: 0g
- Cholesterol: 0mg
- Sodium: 2mg
- Total Carbohydrates: 1g
- Dietary Fiber: 0g
- Sugars: 1g
- Protein: 0g

Ginger Lemonade

Prep Time: 5 mins

Total Time: 10 mins

Servings: 2

Ingredients:

- 2 cups water
- 1/4 cup fresh lemon juice
- 2 tablespoons honey or maple syrup
- 1 tablespoon grated ginger
- Ice cubes
- Lemon slices for garnish (optional)
- Fresh mint leaves for garnish (optional)

Directions:

1. In a saucepan, combine water, fresh lemon juice, honey or maple syrup, and grated ginger.
2. Bring the mixture to a simmer over medium heat, stirring occasionally.
3. Remove from heat and let it cool.
4. Strain the ginger lemonade mixture to remove ginger pieces.
5. Chill the ginger lemonade in the refrigerator.
6. Serve over ice cubes and garnish with lemon slices and fresh mint leaves, if desired.
7. Enjoy this zesty ginger lemonade as a refreshing beverage for your fatty liver diet!

Nutritional Information (per serving):

- Calories: 70
- Total Fat: 0g

- Saturated Fat: 0g

- Cholesterol: 0mg

- Sodium: 2mg

- Total Carbohydrates: 20g

- Dietary Fiber: 0g

- Sugars: 18g

- Protein: 0g

Pineapple Coconut Smoothie

Prep Time: 5 mins

Total Time: 5 mins

Servings: 1

Ingredients:

- 1 cup frozen pineapple chunks

- 1/2 cup coconut water

- 1/2 cup unsweetened coconut milk

- 1 tablespoon chia seeds (optional)

- Ice cubes

Directions:

1. In a blender, combine frozen pineapple chunks, coconut water, and unsweetened coconut milk.

2. Add chia seeds for added fiber and omega-3 fatty acids, if desired.

3. Blend until smooth and creamy.

4. Add ice cubes to reach desired consistency and blend again.

5. Pour the pineapple coconut smoothie into a glass.

6. Enjoy this tropical delight as a nourishing beverage for your fatty liver diet!

Nutritional Information (per serving):

- Calories: 150
- Total Fat: 5g
- Saturated Fat: 3g
- Cholesterol: 0mg
- Sodium: 75mg
- Total Carbohydrates: 26g
- Dietary Fiber: 5g
- Sugars: 15g
- Protein: 2g

Turmeric Ginger Latte

Prep Time: 2 mins

Cooking Time: 5 mins

Total Time: 7 mins

Servings: 1

Ingredients:

- 1 cup unsweetened almond milk
- 1/2 teaspoon ground turmeric
- 1/4 teaspoon ground ginger
- 1/2 teaspoon honey or maple syrup
- Pinch of ground black pepper
- Cinnamon stick for garnish (optional)

Directions:

1. In a small saucepan, heat almond milk over medium heat until warm but not boiling.
2. Whisk in ground turmeric, ground ginger, honey or maple syrup, and a pinch of ground black pepper.
3. Continue to heat for 3-5 minutes, stirring occasionally.
4. Remove from heat and pour the turmeric ginger latte into a mug.
5. Garnish with a cinnamon stick, if desired.
6. Serve warm and enjoy this comforting turmeric ginger latte as part of your fatty liver diet!

Nutritional Information (per serving):

- Calories: 60
- Total Fat: 2g
- Saturated Fat: 0g
- Cholesterol: 0mg
- Sodium: 160mg
- Total Carbohydrates: 10g
- Dietary Fiber: 1g
- Sugars: 8g
- Protein: 1g

30 DAYS MEAL PLAN

Day 1:

- **Breakfast:** Detoxifying Green Tea
- **Lunch:** Grilled Salmon with Steamed Vegetables
- **Dinner:** Pineapple Coconut Smoothie

Day 2:

- **Breakfast:** Turmeric Ginger Latte
- **Lunch:** Quinoa Salad with Avocado and Chickpeas
- **Dinner:** Baked Cod with Roasted Asparagus

Day 3:

- **Breakfast:** Ginger Lemonade
- **Lunch:** Turkey and Veggie Stir-Fry with Brown Rice
- **Dinner:** Broiled Tilapia with Lemon and Garlic, served with a Mixed Green Salad

Day 4:

- **Breakfast:** Detoxifying Green Tea
- **Lunch:** Lentil Soup with Spinach and Carrots
- **Dinner:** Shrimp and Vegetable Skewers with Quinoa

Day 5:

- **Breakfast:** Pineapple Coconut Smoothie
- **Lunch:** Grilled Chicken Caesar Salad with Light Dressing
- **Dinner:** Baked Halibut with Herbs and Lemon, served with Steamed Broccoli

Day 6:

- **Breakfast:** Turmeric Ginger Latte
- **Lunch:** Tuna Salad Lettuce Wraps with Tomato and Cucumber

- **Dinner:** Grilled Swordfish with Mango Salsa, served with Quinoa Pilaf

Day 7:

- **Breakfast:** Ginger Lemonade
- **Lunch:** Veggie and Hummus Wrap with Whole Wheat Tortilla
- **Dinner:** Baked Salmon with Dill and Lemon, served with Roasted Brussels Sprouts

Day 8:

- **Breakfast:** Detoxifying Green Tea
- **Lunch:** Mediterranean Chickpea Salad with Feta Cheese
- **Dinner:** Seared Scallops with Garlic Butter Sauce, served with Steamed Green Beans

Day 9:

- **Breakfast:** Turmeric Ginger Latte
- **Lunch:** Quinoa and Black Bean Stuffed Bell Peppers
- **Dinner:** Grilled Mahi Mahi with Pineapple Salsa, served with Brown Rice

Day 10:

- **Breakfast:** Ginger Lemonade
- **Lunch:** Greek Yogurt Parfait with Fresh Berries and Almonds
- **Dinner:** Baked Chicken Breast with Herbs, served with Roasted Cauliflower

Day 11:

- **Breakfast:** Pineapple Coconut Smoothie
- **Lunch:** Veggie Stir-Fry with Tofu and Buckwheat Noodles

- **Dinner:** Baked Cod with Mediterranean Tomato Sauce, served with Steamed Broccoli

Day 12:

- **Breakfast:** Turmeric Ginger Latte
- **Lunch:** Lentil and Vegetable Curry with Brown Rice
- **Dinner:** Grilled Shrimp Skewers with Zucchini and Cherry Tomatoes

Day 13:

- **Breakfast:** Ginger Lemonade
- **Lunch:** Quinoa Salad with Roasted Vegetables and Goat Cheese
- **Dinner:** Baked Tilapia with Mango Salsa, served with Quinoa Pilaf

Day 14:

- **Breakfast:** Detoxifying Green Tea
- **Lunch:** Turkey and Avocado Wrap with Whole Wheat Tortilla
- **Dinner:** Grilled Salmon with Herb Butter, served with Steamed Asparagus

Day 15:

- **Breakfast:** Pineapple Coconut Smoothie
- **Lunch:** Mixed Bean Salad with Lemon-Tahini Dressing
- **Dinner:** Baked Halibut with Herbed Quinoa, served with Steamed Green Beans

Day 16:

- **Breakfast:** Turmeric Ginger Latte
- **Lunch:** Mediterranean Tuna Salad with Olives and Red Onion

- **Dinner:** Grilled Swordfish with Citrus Herb Marinade, served with Roasted Brussels Sprouts

Day 17:

- **Breakfast:** Ginger Lemonade
- **Lunch:** Spinach and Mushroom Omelette with Whole Grain Toast
- **Dinner:** Baked Chicken Thighs with Roasted Root Vegetables

Day 18:

- **Breakfast:** Detoxifying Green Tea
- **Lunch:** Caprese Salad with Fresh Basil and Balsamic Glaze
- **Dinner:** Pan-Seared Cod with Lemon Dill Sauce, served with Steamed Broccoli

Day 19:

- **Breakfast:** Pineapple Coconut Smoothie
- **Lunch:** Quinoa and Chickpea Buddha Bowl with Tahini Dressing
- **Dinner:** Grilled Shrimp Tacos with Mango Salsa, served with Whole Wheat Tortillas

Day 20:

- **Breakfast:** Turmeric Ginger Latte
- **Lunch:** Greek Salad with Grilled Chicken Breast
- **Dinner:** Baked Salmon with Garlic Herb Crust, served with **Roasted** Cauliflower

Day 21:

- **Breakfast:** Green Detox Smoothie
- **Lunch:** Lentil and Vegetable Soup

- **Dinner:** Baked Trout with Herbed Quinoa, served with Steamed Asparagus

Day 22:

- **Breakfast:** Matcha Green Tea Latte
- **Lunch:** Greek Yogurt with Fresh Berries and Almonds
- **Dinner:** Grilled Mahi-Mahi with Pineapple Salsa, served with Roasted Sweet Potatoes

Day 23:

- **Breakfast:** Blueberry Chia Seed Pudding
- **Lunch:** Avocado and Tomato Salad with Lemon Vinaigrette
- **Dinner:** Pan-Seared Scallops with Garlic Butter, served with Sautéed Spinach

Day 24:

- **Breakfast:** Mango Turmeric Smoothie
- **Lunch:** Quinoa Salad with Cucumber, Tomato, and Feta Cheese
- **Dinner:** Baked Chicken Breast with Rosemary Roasted Potatoes and Green Beans

Day 25:

- **Breakfast:** Acai Berry Smoothie Bowl with Granola and Fresh Fruit
- **Lunch:** Spinach and Feta Stuffed Bell Peppers
- **Dinner:** Grilled Tuna Steaks with Soy Ginger Glaze, served with Sesame Broccoli

Day 26:

- **Breakfast:** Strawberry Banana Smoothie

- **Lunch:** Mediterranean Chickpea Salad with Lemon-Herb Dressing
- **Dinner:** Baked Cod with Mediterranean Tomato Sauce, served with Quinoa Pilaf

Day 27:

- **Breakfast:** Kiwi Spinach Smoothie
- **Lunch:** Egg Salad Lettuce Wraps with Sliced Avocado
- **Dinner:** Grilled Salmon with Lemon Dill Sauce, served with Steamed Asparagus

Day 28:

- **Breakfast:** Pineapple Coconut Chia Pudding
- **Lunch:** Greek Yogurt Parfait with Mixed Berries and Almonds
- **Dinner:** Baked Tilapia with Lemon Garlic Butter, served with Roasted Brussels Sprouts

Day 29:

- **Breakfast:** Mango Turmeric Smoothie Bowl with Coconut Flakes and Chia Seeds
- **Lunch:** Lentil Soup with Carrots, Celery, and Spinach
- **Dinner:** Grilled Shrimp Skewers with Pineapple and Bell Peppers, served with Brown Rice

Day 30:

- **Breakfast:** Berry Protein Smoothie with Greek Yogurt
- **Lunch:** Quinoa and Black Bean Salad with Avocado Dressing
- **Dinner:** Baked Chicken Thighs with Roasted Root Vegetables

CONCLUSION

In conclusion, the journey through crafting a 30-day meal plan tailored for individuals following a Fatty Liver Diet has been both enlightening and rewarding. Throughout this process, we've explored a diverse array of recipes spanning breakfast, lunch, dinner, snacks, desserts, seafood dishes, and beverages, all carefully curated to support liver health and overall well-being.

The cornerstone of this meal plan is the emphasis on nutrient-rich, whole foods, including plenty of fruits, vegetables, lean proteins, whole grains, and healthy fats. By incorporating ingredients known for their liver-supportive properties, such as leafy greens, berries, fatty fish, nuts, seeds, and turmeric, we've aimed to create meals that not only taste delicious but also nourish the body from within.

The breakfast options, from vibrant smoothies to hearty chia seed puddings, provide a nutritious start to the day, packed with antioxidants, fiber, and essential vitamins and minerals. These morning meals set the tone for balanced eating habits throughout the day, helping to stabilize blood sugar levels and promote satiety.

For lunch and dinner, we've explored a variety of satisfying and flavorful dishes, ranging from comforting soups and salads to hearty main courses featuring lean proteins like chicken, fish, and legumes. These meals showcase the versatility of wholesome ingredients and demonstrate that healthy eating can be both delicious and satisfying.

Snacks and desserts are not overlooked in this meal plan, offering guilt-free indulgences that are both tasty and supportive of liver health. Whether it's a refreshing smoothie, a nutrient-packed yogurt parfait, or a satisfying snack bar made with wholesome ingredients, there are plenty of options to satisfy cravings while staying on track with dietary goals.

Seafood dishes take center stage in this meal plan, with recipes featuring omega-3-rich fish like salmon, trout, tuna, and mackerel. These meals provide essential fatty acids that support heart health, reduce inflammation, and may even help protect against liver disease.

Lastly, the beverage options offer refreshing and hydrating choices that complement the meal plan's overall focus on health and wellness. From antioxidant-packed green teas to nutrient-dense smoothies and hydrating coconut water, there's a beverage to suit every taste and preference.

In crafting this meal plan, our goal has been to provide a roadmap for individuals looking to support their liver health and improve their overall quality of life through mindful eating. By embracing whole, nutrient-dense foods and adopting healthy eating habits, we have the power to nourish our bodies, boost our energy levels, and protect our health for years to come.

As the ancient Greek physician Hippocrates famously said, "Let food be thy medicine and medicine be thy food." This timeless wisdom reminds us of the profound impact that our dietary choices can have on our health and well-being. With each meal we eat, we have the opportunity to nourish our bodies and cultivate vibrant health from the inside out. So let us embrace the power of wholesome, nutrient-rich foods and take proactive steps towards a healthier, happier future.